Super Foods
for SENIORS®

Publisher's Note

The editors of FC&A have taken careful measures to ensure the accuracy and usefulness of the information in this book. While every attempt was made to assure accuracy, some Web sites, addresses, telephone numbers, and other information may have changed since printing.

This book is intended for general information only. It does not constitute medical advice or practice. We cannot guarantee the safety or effectiveness of any treatment or advice mentioned. Readers are urged to consult with their health care professionals and get their approval before undertaking therapies suggested by information in this book, keeping in mind that errors in the text may occur as in all publications and that new findings may supercede older information.

> *Without faith it is impossible to please Him, for he who comes to God must believe that He is and that He is a rewarder of those who seek Him.*
>
> *Hebrews 11:6*

Contents

Contents

Contents

Contents

Blues busters

15 foods to lift your spirits

It's easy to get the blues. That may be why feeling down emotionally has inspired such great blues music. Be careful though. The music may fool you into thinking it's just as easy to snap out of the blues and get back to normal.

Like the song from Porgy and Bess says, "It Ain't Necessarily So." The blues are an early stage of depression, and depression can be a complicated situation. It can be a symptom of another condition, or it can be a serious disease all by itself.

Mild depression may be a signal you're not eating right. Even gentle mood changes can be linked to bad eating habits. Shortages of B vitamins, iron, selenium, magnesium, and vitamin C will all bring on the blues. Serotonin, made from the amino acid tryptophan, is an important mood regulator.

As you get older, you don't always absorb some of these nutrients as well as you used to. Aches, pains, illnesses, and changes in your life also can make you an easy target for the blues.

Feeling depressed may be more common when you're older, but it's still not normal. If you feel sad, worried, tired, or irritable for more than two weeks, get help from your doctor, friends, or family.

And watch what you eat. It can help with your recovery and may even prevent the blues in the first place.

1 **Feel good from the folate in pinto beans.** Experts know depression gets worse when you don't have enough folate in your body, and your outlook is brighter when you get plenty of this important B vitamin. A good way to keep your folate level up is to eat pinto beans, the most popular dried bean in the United States. They are among the best natural sources of folate — a cup of pinto beans has almost 75 percent of the amount you need every day. They also contain the brain boosters magnesium and thiamin.

2   **Test tasty tips of asparagus.** Gardeners know one of the first signs of spring is the tender shoots of this delicious vegetable poking through the ground. And this veggie bursts with folate as well. Scientists don't know exactly why it helps chase the blues away, but folate does help your body make serotonin, a neurotransmitter that produces feelings of calmness and contentment. Folate also works closely with vitamin B12 to help you avoid depression.

Cereal	Vitamin B12 (mg/cup)	Folate (mg/cup)	Thiamin (mg/cup)	Vitamin B6 (mg/cup)
RDA-Women over 50	.1	.4	1.1	1.5
Whole Grain Total	.1	1.0	2.8	3.8
Special K	.1	.67	.5	2.0
Wheat Bran Flakes	.1	.9	2.1	2.0
Product 19	.1	.67	1.5	2.0
Total Raisin Bran	.1	.67	1.5	2.0

3 **Snack on sardines for a clear mind.** These little fish are loaded with vitamin B12, which helps your body manufacture the chemicals that help carry messages between your nerves and brain. You can suffer memory loss, depression, and other mood disorders when you don't have enough B12. Women with low levels of B12 are twice as likely to develop severe depression. A recent study found that one in four seriously depressed women were B12 deficient. Just 3 or 4 ounces of sardines will more than satisfy your daily vitamin B12 requirement. You'll also get protein, omega-3 fatty acids, calcium, and vitamin D. But watch out if you're counting calories and cholesterol. Sardines are rich in those, too.

Herb may help mild depression

St. John's wort is the most prescribed antidepressant in Germany, but it's more of a folk remedy in the United States since it is not approved by the U.S. Food and Drug Administration. The American College of Physicians lists the herb as an option for short-term treatment of mild to moderate depression. Studies do not support it as an effective treatment for severe major depression.

4 **Boost your brain with a baked potato.** Folate and B12 aren't the only B vitamins you need to keep your mind working right. High rates of depression are also linked to a lack of vitamin B6 and thiamin. B6 helps balance certain brain chemicals, keeping your emotions on an even keel, and thiamin helps nerve signals travel from your brain to other parts of your body. A baked potato is an ideal way to get these important nutrients along with others like vitamin C, iron, folate, niacin, and potassium. Potatoes are naturally low in sodium, saturated fat, and cholesterol. Just don't be tempted to load up with a lot of salt and rich toppings.

The chart below shows the vast difference in calories, fat, and other nutrients in just two tablespoons of various baked potato toppings.

	Butter	Low-fat Sour Cream	Low-fat Cottage Cheese	Low-fat Yogurt	Salsa
Calories	200	40	20	19	9
Fat	23 g	4 g	.3 g	.5 g	.1 g
Protein	.2 g	.8 g	3.5 g	1.6 g	.5 g
Cholesterol	60 mg	12 mg	1 mg	2 mg	0 mg
Sodium	161 mg	12 mg	115 mg	21 mg	198 mg
Calcium	7 mg	31 mg	17 mg	56 mg	9 mg

5 Live happy with liver. Perhaps it was the way your mother prepared it that made you dislike liver as a child. But then you had some that was fixed a little differently and loved it, or maybe you discovered that chicken livers make great munchies. Whatever the reason you eat it, liver can really raise your spirits because it's loaded with B vitamins that help your brain work better. It has healthy doses of niacin, folate, and B6, and just one slice of braised beef liver will give you eight times your daily requirement of vitamin B12. Just be careful if you have to watch your cholesterol. Organ meats such as liver are especially high in cholesterol.

6 **Grill salmon to balance your brain.** You may think it's the juicy good taste of grilled salmon that cheers you up, but there's more to it than that. Salmon and other fish that live in cold, deep water are full of omega-3 fatty acids, which play a major role in the way your brain functions. Researchers have found that depressed people have less omega-3 than healthy people. They believe omega-3 can actually help drive away depression because it helps slow down overactive brain signals set off by omega-6 fatty acids. Your body needs omega-6, but trouble arises when these fatty acids overpower the omega-3. You get plenty of omega-6 from meat and vegetable oils, so it's important to balance them out by eating salmon and other sources of omega-3. Too little omega-3 also signals you're low on serotonin, which can lead to serious problems such as depression and violence.

TIP
Buying

Don't buy just any old cooking oil if you want to keep your essential fatty acids in balance. Canola oil has more omega-3 fatty acids than other oils, so look for it in cooking oil, salad dressings, and margarine. Corn, soybean, sunflower, and safflower oils have more omega-6 fatty acids.

7 **See a brighter future with sugar beets.** Sugar beets may someday be your ticket to a brighter tomorrow, based on a recent animal study by Harvard Medical School doctors. They found that a diet of omega-3 fatty acids and uridine, a substance that comes from sugar beets and sugar beet molasses, produced the same antidepressant effects in rats as depression drugs like Prozac. The benefits of

New!

Here is a cheerful way to get some extra omega-3 fatty acids — eat sushi served in brightly colored wraps made from familiar vegetables and fruits instead of the traditional seaweed. The USDA's Agricultural Research Service is experimenting with the new product, made from ingredients like spinach, carrot-ginger, tomato-basil, and peach.

omega-3 — found in fatty fish, walnuts, and flaxseed — are well-known for depression, but uridine has not been clinically tested on people. Further research, however, may make it an important solution for the blues in the future.

8 **Eat clams and be happy.** Do you know the saying "happy as a clam?" Well, clams have good reason not to have the blues. They are full of iron, which you need to prevent iron-deficiency anemia. More than 2 billion people have this condition, and a sour mood is one of its major symptoms. Other signs of anemia are pale skin, sluggishness, and trouble concentrating. If you suspect you're anemic, see your doctor. If he recommends getting more iron in your diet, put clams on your grocery list. One 3-ounce serving of steamed clams contains more than your daily requirement of iron. It also has nearly 19 milligrams of vitamin C, which helps your body absorb the iron. Your anemia could stem from a B-vitamin deficiency, and clams are good for that, too. One serving of clams has 14 times your daily requirement for vitamin B12.

9 **Pep up with sweet peppers.** Depression is one of the first symptoms of a vitamin C deficiency, but you can keep your C level up by eating plenty of sweet peppers. Both red and green peppers are loaded with it, and

red sweet peppers have more vitamin C than just about anything else you can eat. Even a slight lack of vitamin C can rob
you of your feeling of well-being. Your brain needs it to produce serotonin, a chemical that makes you feel good and helps
you sleep. Without enough serotonin, you may feel tired and
sluggish. Lack of iron can make you feel the same way, and
vitamin C also helps you absorb iron better.

10 **Drown your blues in a bowl of gumbo.** A magnesium deficiency can bring on low moods,
tiredness, confusion, and lack of appetite — all
symptoms of depression and the blues. Although your body
stores less than 2 ounces of magnesium, you need this vital
mineral for more than 300 life-sustaining processes. One good
way to keep up your magnesium level is to add okra to your
diet. Okra is a southern favorite most famous as an ingredient
in gumbo. This is a Cajun treat made up of vegetables, spices,
and chicken, seafood, or andouille sausage. You can also use
okra as a thickener for soups and stews, boiled by itself or with
tomatoes. Okra and magnesium become more important as
you get older, too. Studies show magnesium absorption at age
70 is only about 65 percent of what it was at age 30. Okra also
is a good source of folate, thiamin, and vitamin C — all nutrients that help keep your mind and mood strong.

11 **Seek serenity from whole-grain bread.** Scientists
have noticed that people with high amounts of
the trace mineral selenium tend to be more cheerful and confident than people with low amounts. Selenium
tends to make you feel more alert and less anxious, especially
when you're low on energy. An easy way to keep your selenium levels up is to choose foods made from whole grains
whenever possible. Two slices of whole-grain bread will give

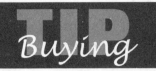

Buying

Make sure you're really getting whole-grain bread and not caramel-colored white bread. The first word on the nutrition label should be "whole" to guarantee you're getting all the nutrition of whole grain.

you almost a third of your daily requirement of selenium.

12 Choose cottage cheese for an upbeat attitude. Researchers know depression goes up when you don't get enough protein. It's one of the nutrients that fuels your body and gives you energy. When you don't get enough, you can run out of gas mentally as well as physically. Symptoms include exhaustion, irritability, forgetfulness, and depression. Cottage cheese is one of your best non-meat sources of protein, so try mixing it with some fruit or vegetables for a meal or snack. This versatile treat is also a good source of blues-chasers selenium and vitamin B12. Just make sure you choose low-fat or nonfat cottage cheese. If not, you'll risk other health problems from high amounts of saturated fat and sodium.

13 Let Cajun rice lift your spirits. The complex carbohydrates in Cajun favorites red beans and rice and Hoppin' John — a combination of black-eyed peas and rice — can help you chase the blues away. They raise the amount of tryptophan, the amino acid your body uses to make serotonin, in your brain. Research shows carbohydrate-rich diets work to lower stress and depression, and complex carbs have a lasting mood-lifting effect. They also boost your levels of vitamins, minerals, and fiber.

14 **Talk turkey about tryptophan.** Tryptophan is an essential amino acid found in turkey and is important in making serotonin, a chemical that helps you feel calm and relaxed. Serotonin also helps regulate your appetite and your sleep cycle. Most antidepressants help you feel better by increasing the amount of serotonin in your brain. Because other amino acids tend to crowd out tryptophan in your bloodstream, you need carbohydrates to help get this important blues buster to your brain. So eat some fruit, vegetables, or grains with your turkey leg for the best feel-good effect.

> Learn more about tryptophan and serotonin and how they affect your mood in *The food-mood connection* feature section on page 10.

15 **Eat an ear of corn when you hear the blues.** You may be down in the dumps because you're not sleeping well, and you may not be sleeping well because your body is low on melatonin. As you get older, you produce less of this important hormone that regulates sleep cycles. Melatonin is manufactured in your brain from serotonin, but you can also get it into your body by eating certain foods, like sweet corn, oats, cherries, and bananas. Experts suggest you include these and other melatonin-rich foods in your diet if you have trouble sleeping.

A Closer Look
The food-mood connection

Feeling down in the dumps? Maybe it's something you ate. Or didn't eat.

Food plays an important role in determining your mood. Just think of the last time you ate an ice cream cone or a chocolate treat. You're probably smiling already. Sometimes a little pick-me-up is all you need.

Of course, sometimes you need more. If you suffer from depression, you can't just magically eat it away. It's a serious medical condition that often requires a doctor's care.

Get to the root of the problem

What causes depression? Experts are not entirely sure. It may stem from a chemical imbalance in your brain. Often it's genetic, which means you inherited it from your parents. But major events, like a death in the family, divorce, loss of job, or major illness, can also spark depression. So can some medications for other conditions.

Women, perhaps because of hormonal changes involved with menstruation, pregnancy, and menopause, experience depression twice as often as men.

Seniors are especially at high risk for depression. In fact, people older than 65 are four times more likely to suffer from depression than younger ones. However, they do not always display the classic signs (*see box*). They may complain of aches and pains or seem confused, agitated, or irritable.

Regardless of its cause, depression demands treatment. You can't just "snap out of it." Without treatment, depression can last for weeks, months, or years. Fortunately, most people improve with the right treatment.

Before taking any other steps, make sure you get a good diagnostic evaluation that includes a thorough physical examination.

Your doctor may suggest proven treatments, including psychotherapy and antidepressant medication.

Danger signs of depression

Look for these clues if you think you or someone you know may be depressed.

▶ **Persistent sad, anxious, or "empty" mood**

▶ **Feelings of hopelessness, pessimism, or worthlessness**

▶ **Loss of interest in hobbies and activities that were once enjoyed, including sex**

▶ **Insomnia or oversleeping**

▶ **Appetite and/or weight loss or overeating and weight gain**

▶ **Decreased energy, fatigue**

▶ **Thoughts of death or suicide**

▶ **Restlessness, irritability**

▶ **Difficulty concentrating, making decisions**

▶ **Persistent physical symptoms that do not respond to treatment**

Fill up on the right foods

Although depression requires serious treatment, eating the proper foods may help as well. The following powerhouse nutrients can affect your mood and help ward off depression.

▸ **Omega-3 fatty acids.** Studies show that the essential fats in fish — called docosahexaenoic acid (DHA) and eicosapentaenoic acid (EPA) — can help drive away depression. That's because they affect neurotransmitters, your brain's Pony Express riders that carry messages from cell to cell. Neurotransmitters have an easier time wriggling through fat membranes made of fluid omega-3 than any other kind of fat. This means your brain's important messages get delivered, not denied access by membranes made of thick, hard fat. Plus, eating fish has an effect on your levels of serotonin, one of your brain's good-news messengers. Fatty fish like salmon, herring, mackerel, and tuna offer the most omega-3, but all seafood contains at least some.

Food combination boosts good feelings

Many antidepressants work by boosting brain levels of serotonin. You can do the same thing with a combination of tryptophan and carbohydrates.

The amino acid tryptophan is found in turkey, chocolate, dates, milk, cottage cheese, meat, fish, and peanuts. When you eat one of these, combine it with a carbohydrate like bread or crackers. The carbs will spark the release of insulin, which herds other competing amino acids — but not tryptophan — to body cells. So tryptophan has a clear path to your brain.

Once there, it combines with various enzymes to produce a compound called 5-hydroxytryptophan, or serotonin — the neurotransmitter that gives you a peaceful, relaxed feeling.

▶ **B vitamins.** Low levels of certain B vitamins, including folate, B1, and B6 — which works by keeping your brain's neurotransmitters in balance — have been linked to depression. Find folate in most fruits and vegetables, especially spinach, asparagus, and avocados. Chicken, liver, and other meats give you B6, which can also be found in navy beans, sweet potatoes, spinach, and bananas. Stick with whole-wheat breads, meats, black beans, and watermelon to punch up your B1, or thiamin, levels.

▶ **Iron.** A sour mood is a major symptom of a lack of iron. Whether you have iron-deficiency anemia or just an iron deficiency, you may experience pale skin, sluggishness, and trouble concentrating. Get your daily iron from meat, legumes, leafy green vegetables, and fortified cereals.

▶ **Selenium.** People who don't eat enough selenium-rich foods tend to be grumpier than those with a high dietary intake of this important mineral. You can find selenium in beef, poultry, seafood, mushrooms, whole wheat, and sea vegetables.

▶ **Carbohydrates.** Recent popular diets have made "carbs" a dirty word. But eating carbohydrates boosts your brain's levels of tryptophan, the amino acid your body needs to make serotonin, the "happy" neurotransmitter. (*See box on previous page.*) Be sure to choose complex carbohydrates, like those from fruits, vegetables, and whole grains.

▶ **Vitamin C.** This mighty vitamin is vital in making serotonin, so running low can leave you tired and sluggish. Orange juice, red and green peppers, citrus fruits, and dark green leafy vegetables provide plenty of C.

▶ **Magnesium.** Some of the same symptoms of depression, including low moods, tiredness, confusion, and loss of appetite, also occur with magnesium deficiency. Look for magnesium in whole grains, nuts, legumes, seafood, and dark leafy greens.

Take action

Eating the right foods can brighten your mood. But don't forget about these other feel-good strategies.

- **Exercise.** When you exercise, your body produces endorphins, the chemical that gives runners what is known as "runner's high." Think of it as a natural mood enhancer. Exercise is also great for reducing stress and anxiety. In fact, Duke researchers found regular exercise may be just as effective as antidepressant drugs.

- **Try tai chi.** This martial arts technique uses a series of postures and slow, continuous movements to relax and align your body. Melt away tension, depression, anger, fatigue, and mental confusion — all without drugs, doctors, or special diets. This cure builds confidence and self-awareness, too. Look for tai chi classes near you.

- **Listen to music.** If it can soothe the savage beast, imagine what it can do for you.

- **Garden.** The peace, tranquility, and beauty of gardening makes this the perfect activity to lift your spirits. Plus, it's good exercise.

- **Breathe deep.** Practice breathing techniques to relax. Deep breathing and calm thinking reduce your levels of cortisol, a hormone your body releases during stress.

- **Join the crowd.** Participate in group activities. Whether it's a class, volunteer work, or a visit with friends and family, being around other people does wonders for your mood. Just sharing a meal together can help. Remember, you're not in this alone. Support of others is essential.

Overcoming depression is not easy, but it's certainly possible. Work with your doctor to find the treatment that works for you, change your diet to maximize key nutrients, and take some steps to reduce stress — and your future will look as bright as your mood.

Tension erasers

13 foods to soothe away stress

You know the feeling you get when you're truly dreading something. Your heart starts pounding, and your hands get sweaty. That anxiety you feel is a natural reaction to stressful situations. It is nature's way of helping you protect yourself.

When you're in trouble, your body releases adrenaline and cortisol, hormones that prepare you to deal with emergencies. Scientists call this reaction the "fight-or-flight response." Once your adrenaline is pumping, your body heats up to generate all the energy and strength you'll need to get past any obstacles. When all threat is gone, your body rests and recovers.

Problems arise when everyday stressors keep you in this mode all the time. You may even suffer from an anxiety disorder that causes constant, unexplainable feelings of dread. If your body never gets a chance to rest, wear-and-tear will set in. Chronic anxiety can weaken your mind, bones, heart, and immune system.

It may be tempting to turn to food for comfort when you feel stressed out, but stuffing yourself won't make you feel better. Instead, fuel up on foods that help soothe your body and raise your mood.

1 **Snack on strawberries.** You don't have to take tranquilizers to make yourself feel calmer. Strawberries can reduce stress and calm anxiety by giving you a surge of dopamine, an ingredient in the brain chemical norepinephrine. This chemical controls how well you deal with stress. Although the link has only been shown in animals, it can't hurt to try a few strawberries when you're feeling anxious.

Plenty of rice to go around

At least you don't have to stress about whether you will find rice at the store. Rice is grown on every continent except Antarctica. A single seed of rice can yield more than 3,000 grains, and a healthy rice plant can live 20 years, producing thousands of grains a year. There is so much rice in the world that it helps sustain two-thirds of the earth's population. Isn't it a relief to know you can always count on rice?

2 **Get help from the B in bananas.** Stress and anxiety use up a lot of vitamin B6 — a vitamin tops in banana's supply of nutrients. Don't let little pressures get you down. Replenish your supply of B6. Snack on a banana instead of coffee and doughnuts to keep a bright outlook on life.

3 **Feel nice with rice.** Another B vitamin you need during stressful times is thiamin, or vitamin B1. Thiamin helps nerve signals travel throughout your body from your brain. When you're stressed, your body will go through its supply of this B vitamin in no time. Replenish your thiamin by eating rice with your next meal. Just one cup of rice will give you 21 percent of the thiamin you need in a day.

4 **Beef up your life.** It's OK to have steak now and then. In moderation, beef can go a long way towards easing tension and anxiety. Red meat is loaded with vitamin B12, a nutrient essential for dealing with stress. Otherwise known as cobalamin, vitamin B12 helps your body make neurotransmitters, chemicals that carry messages from your nerves to your brain and back. Like other B vitamins, B12 gets used up quickly when you're under pressure, so make sure you replenish your supply. If you splurge on filet mignon, you'll be rewarded with 34 percent of your daily recommended B12. You can only get B12 naturally from meat, so if you are vegetarian, you may need to take supplements.

B vitamins in a nutshell			
Nutrient	Also known as	DRI	Food source
B1	thiamin	1.1 to 1.2 mg	rice
B6	–	1.5 to 1.7 mg	bananas
B12	cobalamin	2.5 mcg	beef
Folate	folic acid	400 mcg	turkey

5 **Have a helping of turkey.** No one is ever tense after Thanksgiving dinner. Being with family and friends is part of it, but the Thanksgiving turkey deserves some credit, too. This holiday bird is full of folate, a B vitamin that helps your brain process relaxing chemicals like dopamine and serotonin. It's important to get enough folate because your body uses it quickly when you're stressed. So be smart and serve turkey all year round. Just one helping will give you a whopping 121 percent of the folate you need in a day.

6 **Defeat tension with beans.** Beans may also help your mood when times are tough. In one study, participants under physical and mental stress experienced a drop in

Tension-easing herbs

▸ **Valerian** — Once used to flavor root beer, this herb has relieved tension for centuries. Try it in capsules or a therapeutic tea.

▸ **Passionflower** — Brew the leaves and stem of this flower for a flavorful tea that soothes nerves and offers a break from long-lasting anxiety.

▸ **Ginseng** — This ancient remedy may recharge your adrenal gland, which helps you rebound from stress.

▸ **Black cohosh** — Doctors in Germany prescribe this to treat anxiety. Bonus — it helps with symptoms of menopause.

▸ **Ginkgo** — Take this herb to increase blood flow to your brain and relieve tension headaches in the process.

iron levels. Eating iron-rich foods like beans helps restore this important mineral when you need it most. And don't forget that poor eating habits during stressful times can weaken your immune system, making you more likely to get sick. By choosing nutritious foods like beans, you'll give your body the ammunition it needs to fight off the damaging effects of stress — and that may be enough to help you feel better.

7 Sip some soothing chamomile. Drink a cup of chamomile tea to relieve stress naturally. This hot beverage is so relaxing the scent alone may help calm your nerves. You can find chamomile tea in any grocery store, or make your own by steeping the herb's dried flowering heads in boiling water. When they steep, the heads release a blue oil full of chemicals called flavonoids. These chemicals affect the same receptors in your brain as prescription drugs like Valium. You'll feel relaxed right away without suffering the addictive side effects you might from a drug.

8 **Relax with almond oil.** The next time you feel stressed out, treat yourself to a relaxing almond oil massage. As a carrier oil — one used to dilute other extracts — almond oil nourishes your skin with vitamin E. Just add 10 to 20 drops of any essential oil to every 1 ounce of almond oil, and you've got a recipe for the perfect massage. Keep in mind you should never place undiluted essential oils directly on your skin.

9 **Fight stress with wheat germ.** Studies have shown that stress also will rob your body of zinc. One tablespoon of wheat germ has 13 percent of the zinc you need in a day to protect yourself from illness and other damaging side effects of stress. Try adding this crunchy topping to your morning cereal. Or toss some into your pancakes, waffles, and biscuits for a healthy addition to your recipes.

TIP Kitchen

If you ever wondered what wheat germ is, it's actually cut-up flakes of wheat berry. Its nutty flavor makes a great addition to cereals, pancake and waffle mixes, biscuit and bread recipes, and meat loaf. Look for wheat germ in jars in health food and grocery stores. Keep it in a handy place in the fridge for a quick sprinkle on your favorite foods.

10 **Calm down with oranges.** The next time you feel frazzled, eat an orange. This sunny fruit makes a great snack and is full of vitamin C. Your brain needs this vitamin to make serotonin, a chemical that gives you good feelings and helps you sleep. If you don't get enough, you may feel tired and sluggish. Vitamin C also blocks the release of tension-causing cortisol from your adrenal gland. By blocking stress hormones and boosting your serotonin levels, the vitamin C in an orange can help pick up your mood. Just one orange gives you more than twice as much as you need for the entire day.

11 **Fix some oatmeal for breakfast.** Include complex carbohydrates with each meal to keep your spirits up. Researchers at the University of South Alabama found complex carbohydrates stimulate serotonin production and have a lasting mood-lifting effect. Start with the most important meal of the day. Have a bowl of oatmeal or whole-grain cereal for breakfast instead of a pastry. Grains and fruits break down more slowly than sugary breakfast foods. This will help maintain your body's balance of blood sugar and insulin, and it will give your brain a boost of serotonin, making you feel more calm and content. Research shows people who eat a healthy breakfast every day tend to be happier than those who skip it.

	Coffee & doughnuts	Oatmeal & sliced apples
What you get:	feelings of anxiety from the caffeine in your mug of Joe and almost 11 grams of fat courtesy of the doughnut	your body's natural balance of blood sugar, insulin and serotonin
What you miss:	complex carbohydrates for a dose of serotonin to keep you in a good mood all day	coffee jitters in the morning and the 3 p.m. slump that follows

12 **Pour a glass of milk.** Got tryptophan? Milk does. This drink may do wonders for your mood since it has a soothing effect on your nervous system.

Dairy products contain a lot of tryptophan, an essential amino acid that helps your brain make serotonin, the "happy" neuro-transmitter. Your body changes tryptophan into serotonin, which helps calm you down. Other dairy products especially high in tryptophan are cottage cheese and cheddar cheese. Milk also has compounds called beta-casomorphins that contribute to its soothing effects. So snuggle up with a mug of warm milk, and you'll be relaxed in no time.

13 Open a can of spinach. Popeye eats spinach, and he is never stressed. That's probably because spinach is rich in magnesium, a mineral you need during difficult times. A Yugoslavian study found that people exposed to chronic stress had lower magnesium levels, which only made their stress worse. You can't go wrong if you add cooked spinach to your dinner menu. Just one cup has 157 milligrams of magnesium — almost half your daily recommended intake.

Anti-stress supper

Combine tension-easing foods for a meal that will leave you cool as a cucumber. Try this menu:

▶ Main dish — turkey

▶ Side dish — rice

▶ Vegetable — spinach

▶ Dessert — fruit salad made with bananas, oranges, and strawberries

▶ Beverage — chamomile tea

A Closer Look
Healing powers of herbs & spices

Variety is the spice of life — and a variety of herbs and spices can certainly make a big difference in yours.

Herbs and spices have been used in traditional folk remedies for thousands of years. And they still have a prominent place in today's high-tech society. In fact, a number of prescription drugs feature herbs as active ingredients.

Although often lumped together, herbs and spices come from different parts of plants. Herbs are generally leaves, and spices come from the bark, buds, fruit, roots, seeds, or stems. But they both add flavor to your food and health benefits to your body.

Herbs used for cooking, or culinary herbs, include basil, chives, dill, parsley, sage, rosemary, and thyme. While their main purpose is to make your food taste better, they might make you feel better as well. For instance, basil has been used as a cold remedy, and dill may help with intestinal gas. Culinary herbs often come in fresh and dried forms. When using dried herbs, you don't need to use as much, because the flavor is more concentrated.

Spices fall into the same category. Flavor comes first, but good health often follows. Some spices with feel-good powers include allspice, cayenne, cinnamon, cumin, ginger, nutmeg, and turmeric. For example, ginger eases nausea, and turmeric acts as a natural antibiotic.

On the other hand, medicinal herbs such as echinacea, ginkgo, ginseng, and St. John's wort, pack more of a punch. Rather than sprinkle them on your meat or vegetables, you usually take them in pill form, just like medicine. However, unlike prescription drugs, herbs are not strictly regulated by the Food and Drug Administration (FDA). So you're not always sure what you're getting.

Keep this in mind when dealing with drugs and herbs. Just because herbs are natural does not mean they are always safe. Like any medicine, herbal remedies can have serious side effects. Some herbs interact with prescription drugs, either blunting their effectiveness or dangerously boosting their power. Be especially careful mixing herbs with antidepressants or blood thinners. Make sure to tell your doctor about any herbs you take.

Top 10 healing herbs

Sometimes herbal remedies work just as well as prescription drugs. It's one secret your pharmacist can't afford to tell you. Here is a look at some of the most effective herbs and what they are used for.

▶ **Chamomile — indigestion**

▶ **Echinacea — boosting immunity**

▶ **Feverfew — migraine headaches**

▶ **Garlic — lowering cholesterol**

▶ **Ginger — nausea**

▶ **Ginkgo — circulation**

▶ **Hawthorn — heart disease**

▶ **Milk thistle — liver damage**

▶ **Saw palmetto — enlarged prostate**

▶ **Valerian — sleep problems**

Energy boosters

13 foods that will exhilarate and invigorate

Feeling tired can be as simple as a poor night's sleep or as worrisome as a thyroid problem. Either way, you want more energy, and the right foods can give it to you.

Your body needs core nutrients like fiber and protein for fuel, plus others to build cells and manage basic body functions. For instance, you need iodine to make the thyroid hormone thyroxine. Cut it from your diet, and you could suffer hypothyroidism, a major source of fatigue. Iron, on the other hand, builds red blood cells and ferries oxygen to hungry cells everywhere. Eat too many iron-poor meals, and you may end up dragging your feet from anemia.

But eating for energy doesn't stop there. Vitamin B12 helps absorb iron from food and put it to use inside the body. Five other B vitamins are essential in turning the protein, carbohydrates, and fat you eat into energy you can live on. There's even nutritional help for insomnia, leg cramps, low blood sugar, and baffling illnesses such as chronic fatigue syndrome.

So whatever the source of your slump, rest assured these foods are sure to help.

1 **Start off with cereal for all-day energy.** Eating just one cup of high-fiber cereal in the morning could cut your fatigue by 10 percent. Fiber digests more slowly than most food, so it releases sugars and energy in slow, steady amounts rather than a quick burst all at once. It slows

Cereal for Fiber

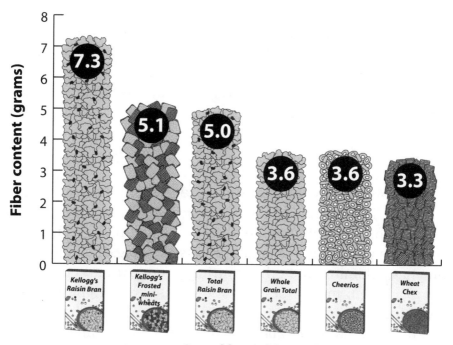

down the digestion of other food, too. All of this helps stabilize blood sugar and even out the energy you get from meals, so each one lasts longer. To get these benefits, experts say compare labels and choose a cereal with at least 5 grams (g) of fiber per 1-cup serving. Take a look at the table for a few quick comparisons. Add blueberries or sliced peaches for even more fiber, and enjoy a bowl every morning for an energy boost that lasts all day.

2 **Liven up with lima beans.** A magnesium deficiency could be the secret cause of your fatigue and muscle spasms. This mineral helps make the sleep-friendly hormone melatonin and control how your muscles flex and relax. Luckily, legumes such as lima beans are loaded with it. A cooked cup of baby lima beans leaves you with 101 mg of magnesium, well on the way to the daily 320 mg needed by women over 50, and the 420 mg for men over 50. Getting more magnesium may particularly help people with chronic fatigue syndrome. So whatever the source of your slump, lima beans and other magnesium-rich foods, such as spinach, whole grains, and nuts, are sure to help.

3 **Wash away fatigue with water.** Feeling exhausted and a little confused? You could be dehydrated. The solution is simple — grab a glass of water. It's the "juice" that keeps your body's chemical processes going. It dissolves minerals, vitamins, and other nutrients and carries them where you need them most. Not everyone should drink eight glasses a day. Gauge how active you are, and pay attention to how you feel. If you're not crazy about water, never fear. Simply substitute an occasional glass of juice, milk, decaf tea, or bowl of low-sodium soup.

| 1 serving of water | = | 8 oz. tea | = | 8 oz. nonfat milk | = | 8 oz. juice | = | 8 oz. low-sodium soup |

4 **Snack on cherries for restful sleep.** Cherries could be the ticket to dreamland, especially if you have trouble sleeping. They're chock-full of melatonin, the hormone that helps you sleep deeply at night and wake feeling well-rested. Some scientists say your body produces less of this hormone as you age, which can disrupt sleep cycles and leave you dragging during the day. Many people turn to supplements, but experts say you can increase your melatonin naturally by changing what you eat. The simplest way — start with cherries. They contain more melatonin than any other fruit studied so far. A handful about an hour before bedtime should do the trick. Experiment with other high-melatonin foods, too, such as bananas, barley, sweet corn, and rice. A banana smoothie or bowl of barley soup makes a nice change from a cherry routine.

5 **Perk up with poultry.** Iron is your body's gold, and like this precious metal, not everyone has enough to live on. Iron deficiency is the most common nutrient deficiency in the world, affecting more than 1.2 billion people. Every cell needs iron to carry oxygen through the blood stream. Too little will leave you weak, tired, and prone to illness. Premenopausal women are most at risk, but vegetarians and people who take non-steroidal anti-inflammatory drugs (NSAIDs) also face a higher risk. Fight back by building iron-rich foods into your daily diet. Lean cuts of meat, including turkey, chicken, fish, and beef, bring you up to speed in no time. But stay away from supplements unless your doctor says otherwise. Too much iron can be toxic.

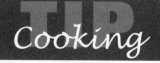

TIP
Cooking

You can triple the iron in food just by cooking it in an iron skillet. Add a vegetable high in vitamin C like red bell peppers to help your body absorb this extra iron.

6 **Quicken your step thanks to quinoa.** You don't have to be anemic — sometimes you're just plain tired. Maybe you need more protein in your life. This vital nutrient is basic energy food. Most people think only meat provides protein, but so do grains. And for that, you can't beat the unique creamy-crunchy texture of quinoa. Pronounced "keen-wa," this funky grain makes a great substitute for white rice in almost any dish. Quinoa cooks in half the time of rice and packs more than five times the protein. Use it in soups, salads, side dishes, main courses, desserts, or even as a hot breakfast cereal like oatmeal. Just rinse it thoroughly before cooking. See how it stacks up against white rice for other energizing nutrients.

Grain	Protein	Fiber	Iron	Riboflavin	Magnesium
Quinoa, 1 cup	22.3 g	10 g	15.7 mg	0.70 mg	357 mg
White rice, 1 cup	4.4 g	0.6 g	2.8 mg	0.03 mg	24 mg

7 **Spruce up on spinach.** Popeye knew a thing or two about the super powers of spinach. Gobbling a can may not give you the strength of 10 men, but it could give you the energy to save the day. The green leaves are loaded with B vitamins, including B1 (thiamin), B2 (riboflavin), B3 (niacin), B6, and folate. This family of nutrients turns protein, fat, and carbohydrates you eat into fuel for your body. The result — more energy. Plus, if you are over 50, just a half-cup of spinach will give you more than a third of the 8 mg of energizing iron you need each day. An easy way to boost nutrition is to use spinach leaves on your sandwiches instead of lettuce.

8 **Savor salmon to beat disease.** Another B vitamin, B12 (cobalamin), teams up with folic acid to help you build healthy red blood cells. Being low in this B vitamin can zap your energy and even lead to pernicious anemia, a fatiguing disease that is difficult to diagnose. You won't have to worry if you eat fish. A 3-ounce filet of Atlantic salmon fills you up with your daily recommended dose of 2.4 micrograms of B12. Experts say older adults may want to seek more since they often have trouble absorbing B12 from food. Only animal food offers this vitamin. For other sources, look to lean beef, turkey, trout, and shellfish.

9 **Balance blood sugar with bulgur.** This hearty whole grain contains chromium, a mineral that helps regulate glucose, or blood sugar, levels by making insulin more effective. People who get more chromium tend to have greater control over their blood sugar levels and are less likely to suffer from diabetes. Plus, chromium supplements in one study dramatically improved the sleepiness, shaking, and other symptoms of hypoglycemia. You may think you get enough, but chances are you don't. A seemingly healthy diet can be high in most nutrients but low in chromium. Your best

Sweet treat for sugar slumps

Bring up low blood sugar with this cool treat, courtesy of the National Honey Board.

▸ Brew 2 cups of green tea and let cool.

▸ Stem and clean 1 pint of ripe strawberries.

▸ Blend berries with 1/4 cup of honey and 6 ounces of frozen orange juice concentrate in a blender until smooth.

▸ Stir in green tea.

▸ Serve over ice.

The honey and other ingredients raise blood sugar gradually, lifting you up from afternoon slumps. Plus they add vitamins and antioxidants.

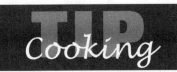

TIP Cooking

Bulgur makes for a low-maintenance meal. You don't need to wash or rinse it before cooking, and you don't even need to stir it in the pot. It swells to more than twice its size when cooked, so just be sure to use a large enough pot.

bet — include whole grains like bulgur as well as nuts, asparagus, cheese, or mushrooms — all rich in this mineral.

10 **Boost thyroid by adding salt.** You've cut back on salt to ease up on your heart, but now you feel tired all the time. You could be suffering from low thyroid, thanks to an iodine deficiency. Most Western countries add iodine to their salt to prevent just such a shortage, and most Westerners eat plenty of salt. But more and more people are cutting back for health reasons. Reducing salt intake is still a great idea. Just use iodized salt when you do sprinkle it on. If you're on a no-salt diet, turn to whole foods like seafood, sweet potatoes, carrots, and even spinach for iodine.

11 **Serve up sweet potatoes.** More iodine won't do you any good without plenty of vitamin A to go with it. Vitamin A helps your thyroid absorb iodine properly. Getting enough is easy. It's abundant in orange vegetables like sweet potatoes. In fact, a single, mid-sized sweet potato gives you 1,096 micrograms (mcg) of vitamin A, more than

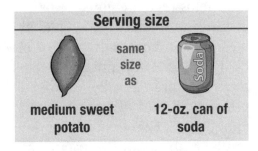

Serving size

medium sweet potato — same size as — 12-oz. can of soda

the 900 mcg a day the government recommends for men over 50, or the 700 mcg suggested for older women. Sweet potatoes are heart-friendly, too, with no saturated fat or cholesterol, but lots of vitamin C.

12 **Go nuts.** The list of nutrients you need for a healthy thyroid keeps getting longer. Now add selenium, an antioxidant mineral that helps the thyroid use iodine and may guard it from free radical damage. A single Brazil nut will fill your selenium bill for a whole day. One nut boasts about 68 mcg of selenium, topping the 55 mcg the USDA suggests adults get daily. Don't go overboard, though. These Brazilian bad boys are high in fat. Settle for snacking on a few in place of greasy potato chips. Look for low-sodium varieties if you are salt-sensitive.

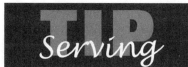

TIP
Serving

Put Brazil nuts and other tough-shelled nuts in a bowl of water, cover, and microwave on high until the water boils. Let cool, then drain. Those stubborn shells should now crack open easily.

13 **Fight chronic fatigue with chicken of the sea.** Everyone feels tired sometimes, but if you have had persistent fatigue for more than six months, you may have chronic fatigue immune dysfunction syndrome (CFIDS). Experts aren't sure what causes it, but they do know most people with CFIDS carry a form of the herpes virus that causes cold sores and mouth ulcers. Arginine, an amino acid in food, helps the virus reproduce. But lysine, another amino acid, may stop your body from absorbing arginine. That means eating more lysine could possibly ease your symptoms. Tuna may be one ticket to more energy. Experts suggest 1 to 2 grams (g) of lysine daily to combat this condition, and one can of drained tuna delivers 3.7 g of lysine, more than enough. Be sure to buy it packed in water, not oil, and look for low-sodium varieties. And don't eat it more than a couple of times a week to avoid potential problems from mercury.

Here are some other lysine-rich foods to eat as well as those high in arginine to avoid.

Lysine — Yes	Arginine — No
fish	nuts
lima beans	brown rice
potatoes	raisins
milk	chocolate
wheat germ	whole wheat
poultry	gelatin

A Closer Look
The 'dirty dozen' — your body's top mood robbers

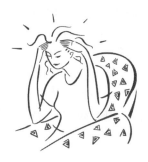

Just as some foods can pick you up, others can bring you down. Keep in mind that these foods are not evil — in fact, many are quite healthy. But they may have elements that work against your body and make you feel bad.

Alcohol. Beer commercials give you the impression that alcohol does nothing but make you happy, young, and attractive. The truth is much more sobering. Alcohol can act as a depressant or lead to aggressive behavior. So, if they kept those cameras rolling, you would probably see those same laughing, fun-loving people crying in their beer, fighting — and waking up with a painful hangover.

Caffeine. A morning cup of coffee seems harmless enough. In fact, caffeine in small doses serves as a pick-me-up. But too much can wreak havoc with your mood and ability to sleep. It may also play a role in headaches.

Salt. Highly salted foods can cause fluid retention and bloating and can lead to cramps.

Sugar. The sugars in foods like frostings and soft drinks can cause mood fluctuations. You may experience a brief high followed by a low. You may enjoy that doughnut at first, but it can leave you jittery and irritable later on.

Aspartame. Unfortunately, this artificial sweetener — better known as Nutrasweet — may be just as bad as sugar. In fact, research links this sugar substitute to memory loss, arthritis, and migraines.

Tyramine. If you take MAO inhibitors, a common prescription anti-depressant, this amine means bad news. Aged cheeses, processed meats like pepperoni and salami, red wine, bananas, and chicken livers contain tyramine. These foods also crop up on lists of possible headache triggers because they make blood vessels in your brain expand.

Omega-6. While not bad in and of itself, this essential fatty acid can cause trouble if you get too much of it. The combination of too much omega-6 and not enough omega-3 can trigger

---

The truth about alcohol

You may read a lot about the benefits of drinking alcohol — how beverages such as red wine may lower your risk for angina, heart disease, and heart attack. And you may wonder if it would benefit you. The best thing to do is to look at it from all sides before deciding.

Alcohol is high in calories but contains few nutrients, so you may want to think twice if you're watching your weight. Plus it may contribute to age-related problems like cataracts and memory loss and can lead to nerve damage in people with diabetes.

It's important to weigh your health risks and discuss them with your doctor, particularly if you take prescription drugs.

If you decide to drink, be smart and combine it with meals, and do it in moderation. That means no more than 12 ounces of beer or 4 ounces of wine each day for women. Men can usually double that limit.

If you overdo it, you cancel out any health benefits and can actually damage your heart muscles and arteries. Plus you open yourself up to a host of other health problems.

---

headaches, depression, and other problems. An easy way to cut back on omega-6 is to limit corn and soybean oils, margarine, and deep-fried or processed foods.

Arginine. If you suffer from chronic fatigue syndrome, the amino acid lysine may provide relief. However, foods rich in the rival amino acid arginine — such as chocolate, nuts, raisins, whole wheat, and brown rice — undo the good work of lysine.

Fatty foods. A high-fat meal diverts blood from your brain to help with digestion. This can make you feel sluggish. Fats often come with a heavy dose of triglycerides, and studies show that high triglycerides equal high levels of depression.

Gas-producing foods. Beans, broccoli, cabbage, and carbonated drinks may make you feel bloated or gassy.

Acidic foods. Tomatoes, oranges, and grapefruit can cause heartburn, indigestion, or gastritis.

Additives and preservatives. Rather than add to your brain's performance, these little extras, such as corn syrup or artificial food coloring, actually subtract from it.

Remember, foods don't always affect everyone in exactly the same way. But if you feel blue, irritable, or uncomfortable after eating any of the above foods, try giving them up and see if that helps. You have too many feel-good food options to let the "dirty dozen" rain on your parade.

Memory savers

24 foods to keep your mind sharp

Some people think time and the ravages of living just naturally take their toll on your brain. But you don't have to expect or accept such a decline. Your brain is capable of great accomplishments, no matter what your age.

Research has shown that your brain does not have to slow down, and you can help prevent mental problems that often develop later in life, such as dementia and Alzheimer's disease. By exercising your mind as well as your body, you'll be ahead of the game as you get older. Things like reading, doing puzzles, and inventing memory tricks are good ways to keep your mind sharp.

But don't forget to pay attention to what goes into your body as well as your mind. The food you eat really does affect your brain, and poor nutrition will put you at greater risk for memory problems. Foods like nuts and cold-water fish give you lots of omega-3 fatty acids, a form of unsaturated fat that helps improve your brain's performance. And a diet low in fat and calories and high in certain vitamins, like C, E, B6, and B12, has been shown to protect against Alzheimer's disease. Don't forget to drink a lot of liquids as well. Dehydration can also cause memory problems.

If you're experiencing memory loss, maybe all you need is a new, healthier diet.

1 **Boost your recall with asparagus.** The B vitamins folate, thiamin, B6, and B12 are all key players in better brain function. Experts say low levels of B vitamins can result in poor memory and possibly Alzheimer's disease.

People well-nourished with B vitamins perform better on memory tests than those with B deficiencies. And according to recent studies, eating enough folate in particular may significantly reduce the risk of Alzheimer's disease. Researchers think a drop in homocysteine levels could be the key. Several studies have found higher levels of the amino acid homocysteine — also linked to heart disease — in people with Alzheimer's. Make asparagus part of your memory-strengthening diet. One cup of fresh asparagus takes care of 17 percent of your folate needs for the day and is a good source of other B vitamins as well. See the following table.

Asparagus & B vitamins	
B vitamin	**Amount/cup**
Folate	69.7 mcg
Thiamin	0.2 mg
Riboflavin	0.2 mg
Niacin	1.3 mg
B6	0.1 mg

2 **Make mustard your condiment of choice.** Especially yellow mustard. That bright color comes from the spice turmeric, which is full of phenolic compounds known as curcuminoids. Animal and cellular studies have found these compounds may help prevent or improve the symptoms of Alzheimer's disease (AD). Although scientists are not sure what causes Alzheimer's, they believe the protein beta-amyloid plays a large role because they have found excessive amounts, called plaques, in the brains of AD sufferers.

Curcumin may block these plaques from forming, as well as remove the amyloid plaque itself. So don't feel guilty about slathering extra mustard on your sandwich — you may help your brain in the long run.

3 **Protect brain health with almonds.** They're packed with omega-3 fatty acids, a form of unsaturated fat that helps improve memory and mental performance and may defend against Alzheimer's. What's more, the almond is a rich source of vitamin E, another memory enhancer. New research has found almonds also contain substances that act like cholinesterase inhibitors, which are drugs used to treat Alzheimer's. A study on animals eating an almond-rich diet showed they performed better on memory tests than those on a regular diet. Their brains also showed fewer Alzheimer's-related plaques. A handful a day of these delicious nuts may be all it takes. Munch a few while working a crossword for a double dose of brain tonic.

> **TIP**
> *Cooking*
>
> You may have heard the old saying "rosemary is for remembrance." It has an element of truth to it. Rosemary is full of antioxidants that will keep your memory sharp as a tack. This pungent herb is especially tasty on chicken and pork and can liven up sauces as well. When you reach for your seasonings, remember rosemary.

4 **Mend your mind with apricots.** This fruit's golden-orange glow comes from the potent antioxidant beta carotene. Since memory loss and Alzheimer's have been linked to free-radical damage, the apricot's beta carotene protects the brain by fighting these free-radical intruders, and preventing and repairing the harm they cause. In a Dutch study of more than 5,100 people ages 55 to 95, those who took less than 0.9 milligrams per day were almost twice as likely to have memory loss, disorientation, and difficulty solving problems as those who ate 2.1 milligrams a day or more. Three apricots give you 39 percent of your recommended daily intake of vitamin A — the vitamin formed from beta carotene.

5 **Count on cantaloupe to help.** It's full of vitamin C as well as beta carotene. Studies find that low blood levels of vitamin C can impair your memory and mental abilities. A cup of cantaloupe has about 52 milligrams of vitamin C — more than two-thirds the amount women over 50 need each day. Enjoy some fresh cantaloupe with your breakfast for a delicious way to start the day.

6 **Grab an apple a day.** This old stand-by has a potent antioxidant that appears to protect brain cells from free-radical damage, a Cornell University study says. Quercetin may be the magic compound. In experiments with rats, researchers found that brain cells treated with this antioxidant, and then exposed to cell-damaging hydrogen peroxide, had significantly less damage than cells treated with vitamin C or not treated at all. More studies are needed to see if quercetin can truly fight off Alzheimer's disease. But since apples — especially the skins — are loaded with it, why not snack on one every day? It just might be your ticket to a memory-filled retirement.

7 **Power up with blueberries.** Give your brain the nutrients it needs for a better memory. You can even reverse the effects of aging and keep your mind sharp. Do it all with sweet, delicious blueberries. The antioxidants in this deep blue fruit safeguard your brain against free radicals. They appear to slow — and even reverse — memory loss caused by free-radical damage. Some experts believe oxidative stress caused by free radicals is at the root of Alzheimer's disease. Research on blueberries is so promising that the berry's extract is being investigated as a way to improve memory, coordination, and performance on speed tests. Sprinkle a few on your cereal in the morning, and you may sharpen your memory and help lower your blood sugar.

Blueberry — a "star" of good health

The blueberry — a true-blue native-American fruit — was originally called a "star berry" because each fruit forms at the site of a little five-pointed flower. But its deep blue color is what makes this berry truly a star. That color comes from anthocyanin, one of its most powerful antioxidants. The blueberry is such a nutritional powerhouse that a half-cup serving gives you the same antioxidant benefits as five servings of either peas, carrots, apples, squash, or broccoli.

8 **Take advantage of boiled rice.** Exercise, heat, and diarrhea can all cause dehydration, and memory problems may be one symptom. You lose electrolytes when you become dehydrated, and that can cause other serious problems as well. You need these salts and minerals in your blood, tissue fluids, and cells. One way to restore your electrolytes, without buying costly sports drinks, is to try a method used in underdeveloped countries to battle diarrhea. Just cook up some rice, and drink the cooled water left in the pot. The liquid contains valuable nutrients from the boiled rice.

9 **Stave off memory loss with olive oil.** Even a modest amount can keep your brain super-charged. That's because of its omega-3 fatty acids, which boost your brain function as well as protect you against other health problems like heart disease and diabetes. In an Italian study of nearly 300 seniors, those who ate at least 5 tablespoons of olive oil a day tested best on memory and problem solving skills. Olive oil's "good" fat molecules appear to buffer your brain against memory loss by patching up fatty membranes affected by aging. So the next time you're in the kitchen, pour on this "miracle" memory booster, instead of other oils like corn or soybean. Although they, too, have monounsaturated fats, olive oil is the best choice because it contains vitamin E and other powerful antioxidants.

10 **Enjoy a banana for a B6 boost.** If you don't get enough of this important B vitamin, your brain may have a more difficult time making neurotransmitters, the chemicals that carry nerve impulses from cells to your brain. This can lead to depression, shortened attention span, and other problems. Studies have shown that people with B deficiencies score lower on memory and problem-solving tests. Chronic B vitamin deficiencies may also be one cause of serious conditions like Alzheimer's disease. Adding a banana to your morning cereal is an easy way to help protect your memory.

11 **Prevent "mental meltdown" with amazin' raisins.** These tiny fruits are packed with boron, a trace mineral the government doesn't consider "essential," but

41

actually affects everything from hand-eye coordination to long- and short-term memory. Studies have shown that a boron deficiency decreases the electrical activity in your brain, affecting your thinking and motor skills. Try pairing raisins with peanut butter and sliced bananas on graham crackers for a hearty, boron-rich snack.

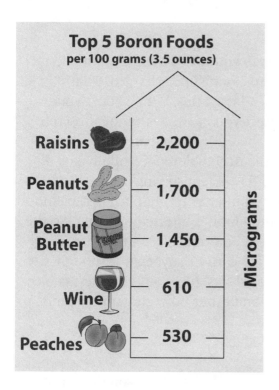

Top 5 Boron Foods
per 100 grams (3.5 ounces)

	Micrograms
Raisins	2,200
Peanuts	1,700
Peanut Butter	1,450
Wine	610
Peaches	530

12 Sample seaweed for something different. Nori — thin, dried seaweed sheets — are used for sushi as well as other Japanese dishes. They are loaded with vitamin B12, an important nutrient in maintaining memory. Just two or three 8-inch square sheets have a whole day's supply. Many older adults are deficient in this vitamin, and up to 90 percent who lack B12 may develop memory loss or depression. To protect yourself, make sure you get at least 2.4 micrograms each day. Trying a different ethnic food like sushi is a fun way to do it.

13 Don't turn up your nose at turnip greens. The secret to staying mentally alert as you age is getting enough vitamin E. Keeping your brain sharp at 70 may be as simple as eating vegetables like turnip greens and spinach, which are chock-full of this potent antioxidant.

Vitamin E helps fight free radicals — unstable molecules that damage your cells. This damage has been linked to cancer, heart disease, and more recently, memory loss and Alzheimer's. A 10-year study of Chicago residents over age 65 found that eating vitamin-E rich foods is more effective than taking a supplement in protecting against Alzheimer's. The research suggests the interaction of the different forms of tocopherol present in natural vitamin E is important. Most supplements use only one form — alpha tocopherol — and studies have shown no association between these supplements and a lower risk of Alzheimer's disease. So focus on getting your vitamin E naturally for the most benefit.

14 **Enrich your diet with spinach.** Memory loss isn't always due to "old age." You may have an under-active thyroid causing your problems. Nutrients like vitamins A, E, and D will keep your thyroid healthy and your mind sharp. Serve regular helpings of vitamin A-packed spinach to protect your thyroid and help keep it in tip-top shape. Steaming is the best cooking method — even better than microwaving — for preserving the vitamins you need. The nutrients don't leach out into the water so you only have minor losses from heat. Or try using fresh spinach as a sandwich topping to reap all its nutritional benefits.

15 **Try an egg-ceptional source of choline.** Your body needs this nutrient to make acetylcholine, a neurotransmitter important for learning and memory. If you want to jump-start your memory in the morning, start with eggs — one of the richest sources of choline. But skip the bacon, sausage, and buttery toast. Egg yolks are high in cholesterol, too, and you don't want to add more from fatty meats and dairy. To keep your cholesterol levels down, eat egg yolks and whole eggs in moderation.

16 **Start with barley for breakfast.** That's another way to beef up your brain power, according to a Canadian study. Subjects began their day with cooked barley and enjoyed a boost in both memory and IQ test scores. Barley's secret to this morning miracle is energy from carbohydrates. Make hot cereal with barley, or look for ready-to-eat cereals with barley listed in the ingredients.

Power up your mind with carbs

A high-carb breakfast can help jump-start your brain in the morning. Try this delicious combination for all-day mental energy.

▸ 1/2 cup oatmeal (27g carbs, 4g fiber)

▸ 1/2 small banana (11 1/2g carbs, 1 1/2g fiber)

▸ 25 blueberries (5g carbs, 1g fiber)

▸ 1 tbsp honey (17g carbs)

▸ 1/2 cup skim milk (6g carbs)

17 **Fight Father Time with the humble prune.** Research shows it can help stave off the diseases of aging, including Alzheimer's and Parkinson's disease. Free-radical fighting antioxidants appear to be the key. When animals were given foods high in antioxidants, they showed less sign of aging on memory tests. Researchers at Tufts University in Boston have measured and studied antioxidants in foods and assigned them a score called the Oxygen Radical Absorbance Capacity (ORAC). Prunes registered a whopping 5,770 ORACs per 3 1/2-ounce serving — more than twice as many antioxidants as the next highest food, its wrinkled cousin the raisin. By adding high-ORAC foods like prunes to your diet, you may lower your risk of diseases of aging, including senility.

18 Go "fish" for brain protection. A study in the *Archives of Neurology* reports that eating fish at least once a week may help keep your brain young. Researchers analyzed six years of data taken from a study of an older, biracial Chicago community. They found that people who ate one or more servings of fish per week reduced their mental decline by 10 to 13 percent per year — the equivalent of being three to four years younger. Although the researchers thought omega-3 fatty acids might be responsible, that association was not shown in the study. More research is needed to determine whether it's the fat content or something else in the fish that helps. But previous studies have shown omega-3 may protect against more serious mental decline like Alzheimer's disease. So adding fish to your weekly menu is definitely a smart idea. It's a high-fat brain food you should learn to love.

19 Make a pot of lentil soup. It's one way to get enough iron into your diet. And without enough of this important mineral, your brain could feel sluggish. A cup of lentils has 2.5 milligrams of iron, more than 25 percent of your daily requirement if you're over 50. Plus they're packed with healthy fiber. Make a big pot of

TIP
Serving

Squeeze a little more iron from your food by sprinkling it with a dash of lemon. Or pair iron-rich vegetables like spinach with orange or tangerine slices in a tangy salad. The vitamin C will help your body absorb the iron better.

Chew on this interesting fact

If you haven't chewed gum since you were a kid, it may be time to pick up the habit again. Researchers have found it could help improve your memory. Several studies have shown that people who chew gum while learning recall the information more easily. Chewing seems to boost your heart rate, increasing blood flow and delivering more oxygen and glucose to your brain. Chewing also stimulates insulin production, which may affect the hippocampus, the area of the brain responsible for memory. Since the chewing action itself seems to be key, it may help to spend a little more time chewing your food as well.

soup, and enjoy several bowls throughout the week to help keep your iron levels up and your mind sharp.

20 Cure memory loss with cabbage. Another fatty acid, phosphatidylserine (PS), may also give your brain a boost. It's a phospholipid, a fatty acid that is involved in communication between cells. Scientists believe as you get older your nerve cell membranes become less fluid and have trouble transmitting electrical impulses. That is one reason older people have more problems with memory and reasoning. PS helps the membranes stay fluid and may also protect cells from damage by free radicals. Several studies have found that PS improves memory and concentration and also relieves depression and stress. It is found in many foods, including green leafy vegetables like cabbage. Enjoy this healthy vegetable stuffed with meat and rice, chopped in a soup or side dish, or shredded in a tangy slaw.

21 **Get into the habit of drinking green tea.** It may help protect your brain from the memory-robbing effects of amyloid plaque, a marker for Alzheimer's disease. An antioxidant called epigallocatechin-3-gallate (EGCG) significantly reduced the formation of those plaques in the brains of mice, according to a study reported in the *Journal of Neuroscience*. Unfortunately, it's possible other antioxidants in green tea may decrease EGCG's ability to destroy amyloid plaque, so drinking the tea alone may not be enough to fight the disease. More research is needed to see if an EGCG supplement is the answer. But drinking green tea on a regular basis may give you a head start in protecting your precious memories.

22 **Jolt your memory with java.** Caffeine acts as a quick pick-me-up when your energy is flagging. Now, researchers have found it may do the same for your memory. Caffeine appears to stimulate the areas of the brain involved with attention and short-term memory. So if you find you just can't remember where you put your keys, maybe it's time for a coffee break. Just don't overdo it. Too much caffeine can result in other problems, and researchers are not sure how it affects long-term memory.

Watch out!

Ginkgo biloba, touted as a first aid for a failing memory, is one of the top-selling herbs on the market. But the jury is still out on whether ginkgo can actually prevent memory loss. You need to be careful if you take it with aspirin, heparin, warfarin, or other blood-thinning medications, since it could trigger bleeding. Talk with your doctor before using this supplement.

23 **Try new recipes with ricotta cheese.** Calcium plays an important role in the connections between brain cells. When you learn and remember something, calcium appears to set off chemical reactions that change connections between the neurons. This complex process is believed to be the basis of memory, learning, and brain development. So getting enough calcium in your diet is critical for more than just building your bones. Cheese is a good source of this vital nutrient, with part-skim ricotta a shining star at 669 milligrams per cup. It's a traditional ingredient in lasagna, but you can use it in other recipes, too, like salads and desserts. Don't be afraid to experiment with this creamy confection.

24 **Relax with a glass of red wine.** Wine has long been touted for its heart-healthy benefits, but recent research shows it may help your memory as well. Resveratrol, a compound found in grapes and red wine, appears to lower the levels of beta-amyloid proteins in the brain that cause the telltale plaques of Alzheimer's disease. Grapes may not have enough concentration of resveratrol to help, but it's possible other compounds in both grapes and wine may help slow the degenerative process. If you enjoy a glass of wine now and then, choose a red variety made with Pinot Noir grapes to reap the most resveratrol.

A Closer Look
Holding on to your memories

Can't remember what you had for lunch yesterday? Maybe you should change your menu. Eating the right foods can improve your memory — not to mention make your meals more memorable. Your personal memory lane may get bumpier as you age, but there are things you can do to smooth it out.

Memory-robbing conditions

No one bats an eye when an older person struggles to remember a name or misplaces the car keys. In fact, the forgetful person may even make a joke about having a "senior moment." That's because memory loss seems to come with the territory of getting older. With age, your brain's nerves shrink, the production of brain chemicals declines, and blood flow to your brain tissue is restricted.

Memory loss also strikes in the form of dementia, a much more serious condition than mere forgetfulness. Dementia is a group of symptoms marked by a change in the ability to think, reason, and remember. It causes serious changes in memory, personality, and behavior. Strokes are one cause of this condition, but Alzheimer's disease is the most common cause, accounting for more than half of all dementias. The hallmark of Alzheimer's is the presence of "plaques" and "tangles" in the cells of your brain. Although scientists have not found a way to prevent Alzheimer's, they have discovered ways to slow the onset and progress of the disease. A healthy diet is a good place to start.

Easy ways to boost your memory

Try these tricks to keep your mind sharp and your memory in tip-top shape.

▸ Solve crossword puzzles.

▸ Play thinking games like chess or cards.

▸ Learn a new hobby, such as woodworking or quilting.

▸ Enroll in night classes.

▸ Find a part-time job after you retire to keep your brain stimulated.

Other conditions that may affect your memory include depression, chronic fatigue, lupus, Lyme disease, head injury, hypothyroidism, and vitamin deficiency. Certain medications for other conditions can also make you forgetful (*see box*). However, memory loss does not automatically come with your AARP membership. You can take steps to keep your memory sharp at any age.

Mind-boosting foods

One easy way to recharge your memory is to rethink your diet. Make sure to choose plenty of foods from a memory-friendly menu that includes B vitamins, antioxidants like vitamins C and E, calcium, iron, omega-3 fatty acids, monounsaturated fats, and plenty of energizing carbohydrates. Cutting calories and trimming fat from your diet will also help, but do not skip meals. Breakfast is especially important to give your brain a jump-start each day.

Herbs such as garlic, rosemary, ginkgo, and ginseng may help with memory, circulation of blood to your brain, or concentration. Others, like chamomile and lavender, can help reduce stress, which is always good for your brain.

Helpful tactics

The right diet makes a big difference in staving off memory decline, but so do these smart — and simple — steps.

- Exercise. Varying your exercise routine provides even more protection.
- Ditch cigarettes and alcohol.
- Keep learning. Pick up a new hobby, or learn a new game.
- Stay in contact with loved ones.
- Get plenty of sleep.
- Listen to music to reduce stress.
- Pop an aspirin a day. Talk to you doctor about this strategy, which might reduce the risk of Alzheimer's disease.
- Take precautions to avoid falls, which can lead to head injuries.

Your memories are some of your most valuable possessions. You can't lock them in a safe with your jewelry, but you can safeguard them with the proper diet and lifestyle.

Medication may muddle your mind

Remembering when to take your medication is hard enough — but it becomes even harder when the drugs you're taking affect your memory. If you take certain medications for high blood pressure, heart disease, ulcers, arthritis, pain and nausea, or Parkinson's, you may worsen your memory as you improve another condition. Many antidepressants, anti-anxiety drugs, and sleeping aids also blunt your memory. Even some cold and allergy drugs can be harmful.

Ask your doctor if the medication he is prescribing can affect your memory and, if so, if there is a safer alternative.

Body-slimming secrets

23 foods that will trim you down

You can win just by trying to lose. Research shows that overweight people who attempt to lose weight will probably live longer — even if they don't reach their weight loss goals. Just picking up the healthier habits of slimming down can help. Keep these guidelines in mind to help you choose the best weight loss plan.

- Eat plenty of whole grains, legumes, and fresh fruits and vegetables.
- Cut back on sweets, refined carbohydrates, processed foods, and unhealthy fats.
- Choose a food plan you can live with for years to come. A successful diet is diverse, so boredom won't drive you to give up.
- Your diet should provide all the vitamins, minerals, and other nutrients you need to stay healthy. Make sure you'll get protein and carbohydrates, too.
- Be constantly on the hunt for high-flavor foods that fit into your weight loss plan.

Plan to lose one to two pounds a week. Your best bet for lasting weight loss is to cut 300 to 500 calories off your daily diet and exercise regularly.

Talk with your doctor before you start a diet if you're over age 65 or if you hope to lose more than 20 pounds.

1 **Tame fat with tomatoes.** Tomato-based foods, like salsa, marinara sauce, and sun-dried tomatoes, can turn simple foods tantalizing, even when you give fat grams the heave-ho. Tangy salsa can replace high-fat gravies and sauces for meat and poultry. It's also a succulent substitute for heavy baked potato toppings, like butter and sour cream. In addition, choose marinara dishes instead of Alfredo or carbonara when eating Italian. And if you perk up dishes with the incredible taste of sun-dried tomatoes, you'll also get the cancer-fighting nutrient, lycopene.

Food	Serving size	Fat grams saved by substituting salsa
sour cream, cultured	1 tbsp	3
butter, salted	1 tbsp	12
Food	Serving size	Fat grams saved by substituting marinara sauce
white sauce, medium, homemade	1/4 cup	6
cheese sauce, prepared from recipe	1/4 cup	8
mild nacho cheese sauce, ready-to-serve	1/4 cup	10

2 **Fight flab with barley.** This ancient grain packs powerful fiber that attacks obesity on two fronts.
According to the USDA, increasing fiber decreases the digestibility of protein and fat, so you absorb fewer calories from them. And, like a sponge, fiber absorbs water and swells,

making you feel full long after you eat it. Soluble fiber, like the kind in barley, even slows the movement of food through your upper digestive tract, so you feel full longer. Add fiber to any meal by substituting barley for white rice in most recipes. Look for barley near the rice, beans, and pasta in your local supermarket. Other whole grains, like oats, buckwheat, brown rice, popcorn, wheat, millet, and corn, can also help free you of unwanted pounds.

3 **Blackball weight gain with black beans.** Lose weight without even trying. That's what 24 men did — even while consuming the same total calories. As part of a university study, these men ate canned beans, a good source of fiber, each day for three weeks. This 50-cent meal helped them lose weight and lowered their cholesterol. Nutritionists have found that fiber can play a major role in weight loss. Harvard researchers found that women who ate the most high-fiber, whole-grain foods gained less weight than those who ate the most refined grains. Eat more foods with more fiber and you might lose weight fast. Get your recommended 20 to 30 grams of fiber a day by eating black beans, fruits, vegetables, and whole grains.

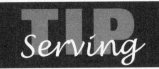
TIP
Serving

Try this scrumptious suggestion from the National Cancer Institute — make a black bean, corn, and bell pepper salad topped with cilantro and balsamic vinegar.

4 **Squash a sweet craving.** Bake a winter squash and spice it up with cinnamon. You'll get plenty of filling fiber and the cinnamon helps the squash taste sweeter. Try this trick with sweet potatoes, too.

5 **Add some zip with lemon juice.** Sun-drenched lemon juice adds fat-free flavor with a healthy dose of vitamin C. You can even buy it in a portable squeeze bottle so it can go anywhere you do. Switch from fatty sauces to lemon juice when you season vegetables, fish, or lean meat. Make a lively, reduced-fat dressing with more vinegar, less oil, plus lemon juice and Italian herbs. Replace butter with lemon juice to rev up the flavor of vegetables. Or top baked potatoes with a whipped mixture of lemon juice and low-fat cottage cheese.

6 **Spice up dull dishes with rosemary.** Plain beans turn interesting when you add taste-boosters, like rosemary, summer savory, or marjoram. The American Heart Association also recommends these delightful seasonings for veggies — chives, cider vinegar, garlic, onion, paprika, or parsley. You can turn low-cal dishes into high-flavor international cuisine with versatile spices.

TIP
Serving

Your body can't burn fat without carbohydrates, so nutritionists recommend that you get at least 55 percent of your total calories from carbohydrates. But when you do need to cut back on carbs, try this. Replace high-carbohydrate spaghetti with spaghetti squash. Cut the squash into two long halves and roast them in the oven — cut side down. Remove the seeds after cooking, and then use a fork to scrape out the "spaghetti."

Cuisine	Key spices
Italian	basil, bay leaves, garlic, oregano, marjoram, rosemary, sage
French	chervil, nutmeg, parsley, tarragon, thyme
Chinese	anise seeds, ginger, red pepper, sesame seeds, star anise
Indian	cilantro, cumin seeds, fenugreek, mustard seeds, saffron, turmeric
Greek	cinnamon, dill weed, garlic, mint, oregano

7 **Block cravings with feel-good oats.** Enjoy the hearty goodness of oats, and you might not crave sweets, bread, and pasta. That's because those cravings can mean your brain has low levels of serotonin, a chemical that affects sensations and mood. Your brain can make serotonin from tryptophan, an essential amino acid found in protein-rich foods. Just eating foods like turkey, dairy products, and nuts can get tryptophan into your blood. But you need carbohydrates to move tryptophan into your brain. All carbohydrates stimulate this serotonin production, but researchers at the University of South Alabama found that complex carbs, like oats, oatmeal, beans, and whole grains, also have a long-lasting mood-lifting effect. These delicious, nonfattening foods can improve your mood and stop you from overeating.

8 **Control hunger with brown rice.** This nutty-tasting whole grain supplies healthy fiber to fill you up. But that's not all. New research may have found a way to learn how to control the "hunger hormone" and crush cravings for good. A small study suggests that hunger-boosting changes in the levels of two hormones that influence hunger could be

linked to lack of sleep. More research will determine whether sleep loss affects how ravenous you get. But why not try some steaming brown rice an hour or so before bed? This grain has melatonin, a natural hormone that helps regulate your body's daily rhythms and promotes sleep. Other foods with the highest levels of melatonin include oats, rice, corn, bananas, tomatoes, and cherries.

9 **Use turkey to carve off fat grams.** Substitute ground turkey for ground beef and you'll cut 5 grams of fat for every 3 ounces of meat. Besides, turkey is rich in tryptophan and protein, which means a turkey sandwich might help boost your serotonin and brighten your mood — a great defense against stress-induced snacking.

TIP *Buying*

Meet the cholesterol-fighting fat substitute made from the soluble fiber in all natural oats. It's called Oatrim. Add it to recipes and it supplies cholesterol-busting beta glucan, yet it has only 1 calorie per gram. Fat has 9 calories per gram. The food industry already uses Oatrim to slash fat. To find products containing Oatrim, look for "hydrolyzed oat bran" in the ingredient list.

10 **Enjoy more water.** Fill yourself up with a tall, shimmering glass of water, and you'll be less likely to overeat, say some experts. But research suggests that drinking about six cups of water a day could raise your metabolic rate — the rate at which you burn calories. In one study, drinking cold water after a meal led to an increase in fat burning in men, while in women, drinking water increased carbohydrate burning. No one is really sure whether simply drinking water will make you shed pounds, but if you choose water instead of other high-calorie drinks, you may be amazed at the results. For a delicious change of pace, experiment with a splash of fruit juice in your water or a tangy squeeze from a lemon or lime.

Drink	Calories	Minutes of brisk walking to burn those calories
skim milk (8 oz.)	83	12 minutes
hot cocoa (6 oz.)	113	17 minutes
whole milk (8 oz.)	146	22 minutes
unsweetened grape juice (8 oz.)	154	23 minutes
cola (12 oz.)	155	23 minutes
vanilla milkshake (11 oz.)	351	53 minutes
chocolate milkshake (11 oz.)	357	54 minutes

11 **Burn more fat automatically with green tea.** It was almost as if they'd discovered how to rejuvenate their metabolism. A group of middle-age, obese women lost twice as much weight as others on the same diet after only two weeks. Their secret? They took green tea extract with meals, which totaled 1,800 calories a day. Scientists suggest antioxidants in green tea, called catechin polyphenols, could help burn more calories. Getting more of these might be the easiest way to lose weight. Talk with your doctor before trying green tea extract for weight loss, but you can start drinking healthy green tea right away. Its caffeine can help boost your metabolism. Green tea might also help prevent heart attacks, cancer, high blood pressure, osteoporosis, and high cholesterol.

12

Snack on chestnuts. A single chocolate chip cookie contains 13 times as much fat as one chestnut, and twice as many calories. So if you need a lightweight snack that won't leave you starving for junk food, chestnuts are worth a try. And don't worry about the high fat content of nuts. This one is different. Most nuts weigh in with five to 10 times as many fat grams as chestnuts. Fresh chestnuts are available from September through February. Pick the ones that feel firm to the touch.

Nut	Number of nuts per 1-ounce serving	Fat grams per 1-ounce serving
chestnuts	12-13	2
pistachios	49	13
almonds	24	14
peanuts	28	14
cashews	18	13
hazelnuts	20	17
walnuts	7	18
pecans	10	20
macadamia nuts	10-12	22

13 **Learn to love olive oil.** This flavorful oil is a beloved food in the Greek diet. Its strong flavor means you won't need much, and its monounsaturated fats help fill you up. But don't just add olive oil to your regular diet. It has 120 calories per tablespoon. Instead, use it in place of other fats and oils. That will be even more fun if you follow a Mediterranean diet. Instead of meals full of fish, chicken, and red meat, include a touch of olive oil to Mediterranean-style dishes full of sunshine-fresh fruits and vegetables and hearty whole-grain breads and pastas. For cheese flavor with less fat, sprinkle a small amount of strong-flavored cheeses, like Parmesan or Romano, over these dishes.

14 **Cast off extra pounds with salmon.** Not only is salmon delicious, it contains a special fat that might help you lose weight. One study found that eating a daily serving of fish high in omega-3 fatty acids helped people lose an extra 4 pounds during a 16-week study. Unfortunately, since recent studies have found many fish to be contaminated with mercury, the Environmental Protection Agency recommends you eat no more than 12 ounces a week of a variety of low-mercury fish and shellfish, like salmon, cod, catfish, tilapia, haddock, sardines, whitefish, anchovies, and scallops. That's either four 3-ounce servings, each about the size of a deck of cards, or two 6-ounce servings. Grill a salmon by wrapping it in foil with a little lemon juice and herbs.

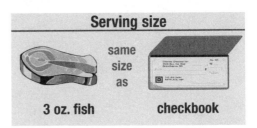

Serving size

same size as

3 oz. fish   checkbook

Energy densities of 3 popular foods			
Example 1	medium apple	calories = 71 weight = 138 grams	71 ÷ 138 = 0.5 (low energy density)
Example 2	tuna fish salad (1 cup)	calories = 383 weight = 205 grams	383 ÷ 205 = 1.8 (medium energy density)
Example 3	milk chocolate bar	calories = 235 weight = 44 grams	235 ÷ 44 = 5.3 (high energy density)

15 **Take the hunger out of weight loss with an apple.** A crisp, autumn apple weighs slightly more than a piece of pecan pie, but the pie slice has six times as many calories. Yet, studies show people tend to eat the same amount of food, regardless of calories. So if you eat foods that have fewer calories per gram, you might cut calories without that starving feeling. The number of calories in each gram of food is called energy density. The more fiber or water in a food, the lower its energy density. You'll feel more satisfied after eating it, and you'll be getting fewer calories. For example, soups have a low energy density because of their high-water content. Try eating other foods with low energy density, like apples, beans, oatmeal, and vegetables. To calculate energy density, divide the number of calories in the food by its weight in grams. The food is low energy density if your result is less than 1.5, medium density if it's between 1.5 and 4, and high density if more than 4.

16 **Punt pounds with creamy yogurt.** Some health experts think your body may hang on to its fat stores because you're not getting enough calcium. Studies suggest dairy calcium might just fix that problem and help you lose weight. In fact, one small study found that yogurt might help all by itself. Yet, filling up on full-fat yogurt or dairy products isn't the answer. Instead, replace other fatty foods with nonfat or low-fat yogurt and other reduced-fat dairy products. Turn yogurt into a baked potato topper or veggie dip by adding garlic, dill, onions, or parsley. For a creamy treat, layer low-fat yogurt and fruit, such as peaches or pineapple, in a parfait glass.

17 **Get more calcium with turnip greens.** Build on your dairy calcium with calcium from a leafy green, like turnip greens or kale. Unlike spinach, these nutritional powerhouses don't contain a lot of oxalates, which keep you from absorbing their calcium. For a super soup, thaw frozen greens in hot water and add them to your favorite vegetable soup during the last five minutes of cooking.

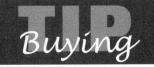

TIP
Buying

Healthy snacks actually cost less than unhealthy ones. Researchers at the National Cancer Institute priced a serving of potato chips at 25 cents and a serving of packaged chocolate chip cookies at 24 cents. In contrast, an apple costs about 13 cents.

18 **Drink OJ, eat less.** Imagine burning as many calories as if you'd been vacuuming floors or walking for the last half hour. Orange juice might be able to help you cut that many calories out of your daily diet. According to a Yale University study, drinking a 200-calorie glass, a little less than two cups, of orange juice a half hour before eating cut at least 300 calories — a net loss of 100 calories or more. Try it for yourself.

19 **Thin the fat with applesauce.** Unsweetened applesauce makes a healthy substitute for up to half the butter or oil called for in your baked goods recipes. Consider the following numbers.

Food item	Calories	Fat
unsweetened applesauce (1 cup)	105	0 grams
butter (1 cup)	1,628	184 grams
canola oil (1 cup)	1,980	224 grams

20 **Throw popcorn at a snack attack.** After-lunch sleepiness can trigger a bout of mid-afternoon munchies. But air-popped popcorn with a tiny dash of olive oil might keep you away from the vending machine. Popcorn can make you feel twice as full as a candy bar because it scores well on the satiety index — an index created by researchers to show which foods keep you feeling full longest.

21 **"Pear" down dessert calories.** After three months on a weight-reducing diet, overweight women, in one study, who ate one pear or apple three times a day lost a little more weight than women who ate one oatmeal cookie three times a day. Pears could be a big help to anyone who loves desserts and sweets. Try eating a crisp, fresh pear in place of a sugary snack. Pears are high in fiber, which helps you feel full longer. Or replace heavy desserts with a baked apple, a juicy orange, or a luscious plum. You could be pleasantly surprised at how pounds melt away.

Satiety Index

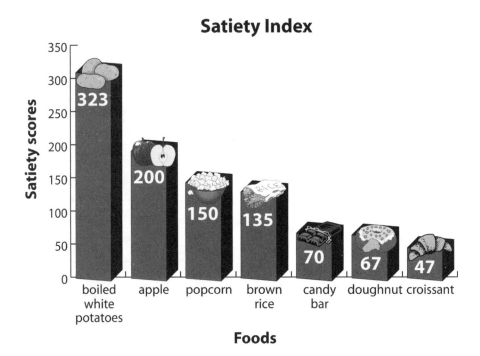

22 **Discover a ricotta stand-in.** You can still enjoy your favorite Italian recipes. Just switch fat-loaded whole milk ricotta with low-fat or nonfat cottage cheese. You'll get the calcium you need, as well as other slimming nutrients, like B vitamins. They help your body turn food into energy and help stave off depression, which could tempt you to eat heavy, comfort foods. You'll also get trypto-phan and protein — two things that may help prevent potential diet-busters, like sleep loss.

23 **Cancel fat grams with cayenne.** You may be in luck if you love hot peppers or spicy foods. A small Japanese study found that men who ate spicy soup or downed a cayenne capsule ate less fat dur-ing the meal that followed. But the soup had to be as spicy

hot as they could comfortably stand. More research will reveal whether this really works, but talk with your doctor if you'd like to give it a try. Unfortunately, hot peppers can make some people ill. If your doctor approves, try spicing up healthy dishes with small amounts of Tabasco sauce, salsa, or green chilies. Start small if you're new to hot peppers and work your way up to larger amounts.

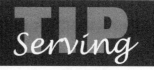

TIP
Serving

Studies show that families who keep fruits and vegetables "in sight" eat more of them. So put a bowl of colorful fruit on your table, and keep cut-up carrots and other veggies in a clear container in your refrigerator.

A Closer Look

Weighing in on weight control

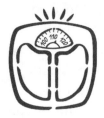

Every year, losing weight ranks as the most common New Year's resolution. Then, 365 days older and a few pounds heavier, people make the same resolution again. But that extra weight puts you at extra risk for health problems, including diabetes, heart disease, high blood pressure, and certain forms of cancer. So ring in the next new year the right way — with a smart, healthy approach to weight control.

Dodge dieting dangers

Everyone wants to lose a few pounds. Unfortunately, not everyone goes about it in a healthy way. Dieting can actually cause weight gain and lead to serious illness of the mind and body. Especially if, like most people, you fall into the pattern of yo-yo dieting — losing weight, gaining it back, losing again, gaining it back again.

Beware of quick-fix promises, "miracle" products, and fad diets. Pills, body wraps, patches, and creams may tempt you, but there is really no easy way to lose weight. If it sounds too good to be true, like swallowing a "calorie blocker" or "fat magnet," it probably is. diet pills can be worse than ineffective — they can be dangerous. Many contain untested and potentially harmful ingredients.

Restrictive diets — like the high-protein, low-carbohydrate Atkins Diet — may help you lose weight, but they often do not provide adequate nutrition. For instance, you don't get enough fruits, vegetables, or whole grains. The long-term effects of such diets, which are high in saturated fats, remain unknown. Plus, it's hard to stick to such a limited diet, so you are more likely to give up and gain the weight back.

Smart steps to safe weight loss

Rather than rely on gimmicks, get-slim-quick schemes, and the latest "in" diet, consider these effective and safe weight-control strategies. The key is to follow a healthy eating plan for life — as opposed to crash dieting a few weeks before the next class reunion. Here are six ways to lose weight that actually work.

- **Eat only what you can burn.** That's the secret to weight control. No specific foods are forbidden. Just remember if you eat that slice of cheesecake, you need to burn off those calories. Your body generally burns 1,800-2,000 calories per day.

- **Control your portions.** Restaurant portions have steadily grown — and so have Americans' waistlines. When dining out, remember you don't have to clean your plate. At home, pay attention to a food's suggested serving size. You'd be surprised how many servings you might be eating at one time. If necessary, use a smaller plate to trick yourself into eating smaller portions.

- **Aim for more plant than animal foods.** Think of meat as the side dish and vegetables as the entrée. Plant-based foods should cover at least two-thirds of your plate. Eat half your usual portion of meat and have two veggies instead of one.

- **Exercise regularly.** Eating less plus moving more equals subtracted pounds. Aim for one hour a day of moderate exercise. It can be as simple as going for a walk.

- **Keep a food diary.** Take note of what you eat and how you feel.

- **Set realistic goals.** Expect to lose about 10 percent of your weight. Slow and steady wins the race. Reward yourself for reaching mini-goals — but not with food.

If you think dieting means denying yourself, think again. Lose weight permanently and stay healthy and happy by eating more, not less. Just opt for foods with a high water content, which fill you up without filling you with calories. Try soups instead of casseroles, and add vegetables to salads, pasta dishes, and sandwiches.

High-fiber foods, like fruits, veggies, and whole grains, also help you lose weight. Much of dietary fiber can't be digested, so it passes through your system. But it also fills you up, keeps you satisfied longer, and may block the absorption of some of the fat and protein you eat. Just changing your fiber intake — without altering the number of calories you eat — could mean losing a couple of pounds a month.

You can eat more and weigh less as long as you make every calorie count. Cut back on added sugars, fats, and alcohol, which provide calories but few or no essential nutrients.

Plan for success

They say failing to plan is planning to fail. That certainly applies to weight control. You have many options, but one worth considering is the Pritikin Plan, possibly the last diet you'll ever need. In less than one month, women and men on this delicious and nutritious plan lost weight without dieting, reduced their cholesterol 21 percent, improved their sense of well being, and felt less anxiety and fear.

The basic elements of this program, which has been around since the 1970s, include a diet low in fat, calories, and salt as well as moderate exercise. If you're interested in how this program can help you, call the Pritikin Longevity Center at 800-327-4914, or check the Web site at *www.pritikin.com*.

Maintenance strategies that work

So you've managed to get down to your target weight. Now what? Maintaining your weight is just as important as losing weight — and often as difficult. But it doesn't have to be. When it comes to taking it off and keeping it off, focus on weight-loss strategies that work for a lifetime. According to data from the National Weight Control Registry, people who have succeeded at losing and maintaining weight limit fast foods to less than once a week, weigh themselves regularly, eat five times a day, and burn an average of 400 calories a day through exercise.

When you're trying to lose weight, you must burn more calories than you take in. But it's important to keep on eye on your calories even after you reach your desired weight. Work off the same amount of calories you take in, and your weight will stay the same.

Fitness fare

18 foods to help you shape up safely

Your body thrives when you stay in shape. You feel healthier, live longer, and resist diseases better when you keep fit. Exercise is also your best bet to take off and keep off ugly, unwanted pounds.

But you have to be smart about what you eat. Since exercise burns up calories, protein, and carbohydrates, you can — and should — eat enough to give your body the proper amount of fuel. But exercise is not a license to overeat. Proper fitness includes a diet that provides most of your nutrients from whole grains, fruits, and vegetables, as few animal fats and hydrogenated oils as possible, and little or no added salt and sugar.

Physical activity also uses more vitamin C, vitamin E, potassium, magnesium, and calcium. Without the right vitamins and minerals, you're liable to cramp up and suffer unneeded aches and pains. And when you work out, you can get away with larger portions of healthy food because you need those extra nutrients. A large orange, for instance, gives you 98 milligrams (mg) of vitamin C, while you only get 51 mg from a small one.

Good nutrition also cuts your chances of exercise-induced asthma, a fitness side-effect that impacts almost 90 percent of people who have asthma and up to 10 percent of the general population. Drinking water and loading up on certain antioxidants may be one way to help prevent this type of asthma attack.

1 **Put whole grain bagels on your table.** You can't do much better for a breakfast treat that gives you energy all day long. Complex carbohydrates like the ones in whole grain products give you the best energy and are also an important source of vitamins, minerals, phytochemicals, and fiber. Complex carbs break down more slowly than the simple carbohydrates found in sugars and highly processed grains. You get longer-lasting energy and more stable insulin and blood sugar levels instead of a sudden surge of power and then a big letdown. Choose foods that have names like these at the top of their ingredient lists: whole wheat, whole rye, oatmeal, brown rice, etc. If the label says wheat flour, enriched flour, or 7-grain bread, watch out. They're fancy names, but they aren't whole grain.

2 **Chow down on pork and beans.** They're the ultimate campfire meal, hot or cold, eaten right out of the can. Not only are they tasty and easy to fix, they also pep up your blood after a day of hiking or other activity. Just one cup of pork and beans has a full day's supply of iron and more than a day's supply of zinc. You need iron for hemoglobin and myoglobin, two compounds that carry oxygen throughout your blood to your muscles. Without enough iron, you feel weak and listless. Zinc is an essential mineral that

Black beans end back pains

Follow an old Asian folk remedy to relieve and prevent lower back problems. Start with a cup of black beans, and soak them overnight. Bring the beans to a boil in three and a half cups of water, then simmer covered for two and a half hours. Remove foam that forms on top. Eat two tablespoons of the beans every day for a month, then every other day for another month. Make fresh beans every three or four days. If your back is better after the two months, keep up the routine.

stimulates activity in many enzymes, including carbonic anhydrase, an enzyme that helps your body get rid of carbon dioxide. A recent study shows that, without it, you feel tired and weak when you exercise.

3 **Treat yourself to a honey pick-me-up.** Try a spoonful of honey in water just before you exercise and again when you think you need an extra boost of strength. Honey has a great supply of natural carbohydrates, your best source of energy. You get about the same power jolt from honey as from glucose, the sugar used in energy bars and gels. The sweet nectar tastes better, though, and is a lot less expensive. Take honey after your workout, too. It helps your muscles recuperate, replaces the extra carbs you used, and keeps up your immune system.

Burn fat before you eat it

You can burn off monounsaturated fat by exercising before you eat, a University of Wisconsin study shows. Your metabolism speeds up and then keeps working on those plant-based fats. It doesn't work on saturated animal fat, though. So go to the gym, then come home and eat olive oil and other vegetable fats without worrying that they're going to your hips. Just don't expect the same result if you have a juicy steak and real butter.

4 **Snack on peanuts, but hold the salt.** Your body burns protein when you exercise, and a handful of peanuts is a great way to get it back. Most sources of protein — especially meat — are full of saturated fat and cholesterol. Peanuts have fat, too, but it's mostly monounsaturated fat, the best kind to have. They have very little saturated fat, and no cholesterol. Along with the protein, peanuts also give you fiber, and they satisfy your hunger so you don't crave other fatty foods. Just make sure you choose unsalted peanuts. They have less than 2 mg of sodium per ounce while a salted ounce of peanuts has a whopping 230 mg. Although sodium is an electrolyte your body needs, unless you're a serious athlete, you already get plenty of this mineral.

5 **Add an energy bar when you need quick fuel.** They come in many brands and flavors, and they all promise to be good for you. Under the right circumstances, they are. A hard workout burns a lot of energy, and these bars are packed with calories, carbohydrates, fats, and protein that will replace that energy. Called — among other things — nutrition bars, protein bars, and diet bars, these little lumps of power were developed to give quick fuel to marathon runners. Now all sorts of people use them to boost energy, lose weight, curb hunger, or replace meals. Ingredients vary widely, so read labels carefully and pick a bar that has what you need. Make sure you'll burn more calories than you take in. Your best energy comes from long-term carbohydrates, not a short-term sugar rush. Extra fat and protein are only needed if you're trying to build more muscle. The more fiber and less saturated fat you get, the better. Many experts believe you don't need an energy bar unless your workout is at

Use apricot oil to soothe achy muscles

Apricot oil is a "carrier oil" for aromatic essential oils that work wonders on muscle aches and pains. Mix these ancient fragrances in an amber glass bottle: 12 drops lavender, 6 drops rosemary, 4 drops juniper, and 3 drops peppermint. Add a tablespoon each of apricot and vegetable oil, stir, and rub into your sore muscles. Better yet, ask a friend or family member for a relaxing massage using this potion.

least two hours long. Use the table below to compare the nutrients in energy bars, a granola bar, and a candy bar.

Nutrient	Chocolate Power Bar	Chocolate BalanceBar	Chocolate Decadence Atkins Advantage	Milk Choc/ChocChip Granola Bar	Snickers Bar
Serving size (g)	65	50	60	35	57
Calories	230	200	260	163	266
Fat (g)	2	6	10	9	11
Saturated fat (g)	0.5	3.5	7	5	4
Total Carbs (g)	45	22	26	22	37
Sugars (g)	18	18	4	–	28
Fiber (g)	3	1	11	1	1
Protein (g)	10	14	17	2	5
Sodium [mg]	95	180	80	70	130
Potassium [mg]	200	160	–	110	184

6 **Eat lean meat after you exercise.** It's a good way to get leucine, a protein building block that repairs damaged muscles. Your sore muscles heal and rebuild faster with this essential amino acid's help. Studies have shown that protein in a weight-loss diet helps you burn away fat instead of muscle, and leucine is the particular protein that gets most of the credit. In addition to fueling your muscles, leucine helps with your metabolism and in maintaining your blood sugar after exercise. A post-workout turkey sandwich would fit the bill nicely.

7 **Peel a banana for a wonderful workout.** Bananas are cheap, sweet, nutritious, and come in their own germ-proof package. They're full of complex carbohydrates and potassium — two key components of a good exercise session. Potassium is one of the minerals you lose when you sweat, and complex carbs are the best way to get energy. Your body burns carb calories faster and easier than fat or protein calories, and bananas have more digestible carbohydrates than any other fruit. It's no wonder many endurance athletes usually have a banana in their gym bag.

Watch out!

Bananas, peanuts, and almonds may trigger exercise-induced asthma (EIA), so be careful about eating them before physical activity if you have asthma or asthma symptoms. These foods — along with shrimp, celery, and egg whites — are the most common causes of food-related EIA. They can kick off an attack that will leave you gasping and wheezing if you eat them even two hours before exercising.

8 **Chew sunflower seeds to keep cramps away.** These tiny morsels are full of vitamin E, which researchers believe is a good treatment for muscle cramps. Studies

75

show this powerful antioxidant works just as well as quinine — and with fewer side effects — to quiet cramps. People with intermittent claudication, which produces painful leg cramps, are usually low on vitamin E. You can get sunflower seeds already shelled and eat them as a snack, or sprinkle them on salads. An ounce of these kernels gives you more than two thirds of your daily requirement for vitamin E.

9 **Drink milk to put a crimp on cramps.** Calcium is best known for building your bones, but it also keeps your muscles moving. Among other things, it helps contract muscles and send nerve impulses. So if you get muscle cramps when you exercise, it may mean you're short on this mineral. A glass of milk is a great place to get more. Just one cup of skim milk has more than 300 mg of calcium as well as 400 mg of potassium — another mineral that prevents cramps. Milk is also an ideal quick source of protein and carbohydrates.

Watch out!

You should get some sun if you want to keep calcium in your body. That's because your skin converts sunlight to vitamin D, which you need to absorb calcium. Too much vitamin D from supplements can be toxic, so getting 15 minutes of sun twice a week on your face, hands, and arms is the best way to go.

10 **Dampen your cramps with plain old water.** Dehydration is probably the most common cause of muscle cramps when you exercise. It also adds to your problems with exercise-induced asthma. You can prevent dehydration if you just drink plenty of water — at least six full glasses every day, and more when you exercise. Plain water is the best hydrator because it gets to your tissues faster than beverages that have to be digested. Don't wait until you're thirsty to avoid dehydration, though. Exercise actually slows down your thirst mechanism, which takes even longer to react as you get older. Keep a water bottle handy, and sip it while you're working out. You'll also help head off heat exhaustion and heatstroke.

11 **Nibble almonds to keep your muscles moving.** These tasty nuts are one of the best foods you can eat to reload the minerals you lose from dehydration. A handful of almonds gives you substantial amounts of magnesium, potassium and calcium — the big three minerals for preventing cramps and making your muscles work properly. Almonds are also packed with the antioxidant power of vitamin E, another cramp-fighting nutrient. Vitamin E also fights asthma and helps your lungs work better. To top it off, an ounce of almonds has 6 grams of protein to give your body more energy for your workout.

TIP
Buying

Keep a bottle or two of a sports drink like Gatorade or Powerade on your shelves for times when you're exceptionally active. These thirst-quenchers are designed to recharge important nutrients and minerals you lose when you sweat a lot. The right food and plenty of water are best for ordinary exercise, but sometimes a more intense workout means you can use the extra sodium, potassium, and sugars in a sports drink.

12 **Pop pumpkin seeds for more magnesium.** It's a handy, tasty way to keep your muscles working right while you're working out. Magnesium helps control how well muscles flex and relax. You need it to ward off both cramps and fatigue. Magnesium also acts as a bronchodilator, which opens up your airways and makes it easier to breathe. You can buy packaged pumpkin seeds, or you can roast them yourself. Scoop out the seeds from your jack-o-lantern, wipe them off, and spread them on a cookie sheet. Coat them lightly with olive oil and roast for about 45 minutes at 375 degrees. Keep them in an airtight container until you're ready for an exercise snack.

Limit EIA with a low-salt diet

People with exercise-induced asthma breathe better if they don't eat a lot of salt. An Indiana University study found that participants who ate about 9,800 milligrams of sodium a day had a severe drop in lung function after physical activity, and those who took in only 1,446 mg a day practically eliminated their EIA symptoms.

13 **Think pink grapefruit and breathe better.** You could be in a lot of trouble if working out kicks off your asthma, but grapefruit may put you in the pink for protection against breathing problems from exercise-induced asthma (EIA). Some research says lycopene protects against EIA, and pink grapefruit is loaded with lycopene.

Although other studies are not so sure about the lycopene/asthma connection, scientists do know people with breathing problems tend to have low levels of lycopene and other potent carotenoids. And lycopene isn't grapefruit's only important nutrient. It's also a good source of vitamin C and vitamin A. You can get three quarters of a day's supply of vitamin C — the main antioxidant in the surface of your lungs — from half a large grapefruit.

14 **Mind the minerals in broccoli.** It's not surprising this crunchy crucifer, which is a good source of nearly all the nutrients you'll ever need, also contains the two most important asthma-fighting minerals — magnesium and selenium. Studies show that people with low levels of selenium are more likely to have asthma, and 90 percent of asthmatics are likely to suffer attacks when they exercise. Magnesium acts as a bronchodilator, helping to open up your airways so you can breathe easier. Add avoiding an EIA attack while you exercise to your list of reasons to include broccoli in your diet.

Eat better and duck drugs

People with asthma who have too many omega-6 fatty acids and not enough antioxidants are liable to have attacks when they exercise. Drugs are the usual treatment for EIA, but research has found that changing the amounts you get of these nutrients may make a difference. By strengthening your diet, you may be able to fight off EIA without medication.

15 **Boost your body with a shot of caffeine.** A java jolt from a cup of coffee or a can of cola might be just the ticket if you're prone to asthma attacks while you exercise. The caffeine acts as a mild bronchodilator, relaxing and expanding the air passages in your lungs, and it peps up tired muscles in your respiratory system. Caffeine also helps some people deal with muscle aches and pain, which is why it's in so many over-the-counter pain relievers. Research also shows caffeine may boost your endurance while you exercise. It seems to work best if you are not a frequent caffeine user and drink about a cup of coffee from one to three hours before working out.

Watch out!

Don't get carried away if you use coffee to give you a workout lift. A cup
or two a day is plenty. Too much caffeine can cause anxiety,
headaches, and upset stomach. It can also prevent your
body's natural pain fighters from doing their job, and caffeine
flushes calcium out of your body.

16 **Squeeze an orange and heal sore muscles.** The vitamin C in oranges does double duty to ease the aches, pains, and swelling you get from a workout. Its antioxidant power gets rid of free radicals caused by injured or inflamed muscles. Your body also needs vitamin C to make collagen, a protein that builds and repairs cartilage, ligaments, muscles, and bones. When you have plenty of collagen, damaged muscles heal faster and bruises go away more quickly. Just one orange gives you almost 70 mg of vitamin C. This water-soluble vitamin is so important, though, that some experts suggest taking a 500-mg supplement before exercising to prevent soreness.

17 **Mix mustard in a cup of water.** Then drink it to stop your muscle cramps. That's a solution trainers at the University of Alabama say works wonders for their athletes. Researchers haven't figured out why it works, but they suspect vinegar has something to do with it. If you've been cramping up on your workouts, take along some packets of mustard. When the spasms start, stir a packet into water and take a swig. If you don't have water available, just eat it straight from the packet. Repeat every couple of minutes until the mustard turns the tide.

18 **Guzzle grape juice when your legs hurt.** You may be suffering from intermittent claudication, which happens when blood vessels in your legs get clogged with cholesterol. Your muscles ache and clench up because they can't get enough oxygen-rich blood. Grape juice seems to make blood vessels more elastic and your blood less sticky, which improves your circulation and eases the aches. Scientists believe it's the flavonoid antioxidants in grapes that make the difference. Research suggests it takes a couple of 12-ounce glasses of grape juice a day to get relief from intermittent claudication. Exercise helps, too, so plan some longer walks. That much juice has 460 calories, and the extra exercise will help to burn some of them away.

Pick pickle juice

Another folk remedy for cramps from the playing fields is pickle juice. Many athletes, coaches, and trainers say a 2-ounce shot about an hour before the game will stop cramping later on. Sauerkraut may have the same effect. Try it before you exercise, but check with your doctor if you need to avoid salt.

A Closer Look
Understanding dietary guidelines

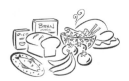

Everywhere you turn, some so-called expert is dishing out new diet advice. Magazines, television, and the latest bestselling diet books serve up a heaping plate of hype — with a meaty side of confusion. Who to believe?

You might try the *Dietary Guidelines for Americans.* Developed by the U.S. Department of Health and Human Services and the USDA, the Dietary Guidelines provide science-based advice to promote health and reduce the risk of chronic diseases through diet and physical activity. They are reviewed and updated every five years, and the latest edition just came out in 2005. Here are some of the new Guidelines' key recommendations.

Veg out. Try for two cups of fruit and two and a half cups of vegetables per day, based on a standard 2,000-calorie diet. Make sure to get a variety of fruits and veggies, including dark green, orange, and starchy vegetables, and legumes. The Guidelines also encourage you to eat whole grains, which should make up at least half your grains, and three cups a day of fat-free or low-fat milk and milk products.

Trim the fat. Limit fat intake to 20 to 35 percent of your total calories, with no more than 10 percent from saturated fats. Opt for lean meats and low-fat or fat-free milk products. You should also keep your daily cholesterol intake under 300 milligrams (mg), and eat as few trans fats as possible.

Choose the right carbs. Load up on fiber-rich fruits, vegetables, and whole grains, but limit foods with added sugars and sweeteners. To prevent dental decay, practice good oral hygiene and cut back on sugar- and starch-containing foods.

Skimp on salt. Aim for less than 2,300 mg, or about one tea-spoon, of sodium per day. Choose and cook foods with little salt, while eating potassium-rich fruits and vegetables.

Curb alcohol. If you choose to drink, do so in moderation. That means one drink a day for women and two for men.

Get moving. The Guidelines stress the importance of physical activity to reduce the risk of chronic disease, manage body weight, and achieve weight loss. Make time for at least 30 minutes of exercise most days of the week. You'll benefit even more if you increase that to 60 minutes or, if you need to lose weight, 90 minutes. It's a good idea to talk to your doctor before starting an exercise program.

You can download a copy of the entire *Dietary Guidelines for Americans 2005* at *www.healthierus.gov/dietaryguidelines*. You can also purchase a copy by calling toll-free 866-512-1800.

Pyramid scheme

You don't need a degree in archaeology to discover the secrets of the USDA's revamped food pyramid. Just go to *www.MyPyramid.gov* to check out *My Pyramid* — a handy companion to the Dietary Guidelines.

The color-coded pyramid takes into account grains, vegetables, fruits, milk, oils, and meat and beans. Click on each part of the pyramid to learn more about each food group. You can even per-sonalize the information by entering your age, sex, and level of physical activity. You'll get a customized list showing how much of each food group you should eat each day, along with tips to help you fit these foods into your diet.

Be physically active for at least 30 minutes most days of the week.

For a 2,000-calorie diet, you need the amounts below from each food group every day.

GRAINS	VEGETABLES	FRUITS	MILK	MEAT&BEANS
6 oz.	2 1/2 cups	2 cups	3 cups	5 1/2 oz.

For more information, go to MyPyramid.gov.

Keep the pyramid in mind when you shop for groceries, and you'll make smart food choices. Read labels carefully to limit saturated or trans fats, sodium, and added sugars and to make sure you get enough whole grains. Grab a variety of fruits and vegetables — the more colors, the better — and remember that frozen or canned ones work, too.

DRIs answer SOS

Still unsure how much of a certain nutrient you need? Look no further than the Dietary Reference Intakes. Established by the Food and Nutrition Board of the National Academy of Sciences, the Dietary Reference Intakes (DRIs) include either Recommended Daily Allowances (RDAs) or Adequate Intakes (AIs) for almost every nutrient imaginable. RDA levels are based on more scientific evidence, but both numbers serve as useful goals.

Sunshine superhero

Do you cover yourself with long sleeves, a wide-brimmed hat, and sunscreen when you're out in the sun? That's great for preventing skin cancer but not so great when it comes to getting enough vitamin D. This vitamin, which your body makes from sunlight, helps you absorb calcium and reduces the risk of bone loss. But chances are you're not getting enough of this important nutrient. In fact, the *Dietary Guidelines for Americans 2005* recommends that older people, people with dark skin, and people who don't get enough sunlight consume extra vitamin D from vitamin D-fortified foods, like milk or orange juice, or supplements. A little more time in the sun won't hurt, either.

Super joint soothers

19 foods to keep you moving

Few things hurt worse than the pain of arthritic and inflamed joints. Unfortunately, it's a common condition, especially when you get older. Almost everyone over age 70 has some symptoms of osteoarthritis (OA), but you can also have rheumatoid arthritis (RA) or gout. All three will give you painful, swollen joints.

Four out of five adults over 50 have some sort of OA, caused by wear and tear on the soft tissue in your joints. As this cartilage disappears, you get painful bone-on-bone contact when you move your joints.

RA only affects 1 to 2 percent of the population, often between the ages of 20 and 40, and women more than men. It happens when your autoimmune system goes haywire, and infection-fighting white blood cells attack your joints instead. Left unchecked, RA can even spread to your heart and lungs. Gout is a type of arthritis that results when your body has problems with uric acid, a natural byproduct of metabolism.

Doctors don't have many medical cures for arthritis. They try to slow it down and control the pain with nonsteroidal anti-inflammatory drugs (NSAIDs) and other painkillers. They also prescribe exercise and weight loss.

But good nutrition may be your best bet to soothe the soreness of swollen and painful joints. The right food helps ease inflammation and repair damaged tissues. It's also vital for maintaining a healthy weight.

1 **Beat arthritis with colorful apricots.** Colorful fruits like apricots get their brightness from antioxidants that can help keep your knees safe from osteoarthritis and defend you against other kinds of arthritis. Apricots also give you a big boost of potassium, which is important if you take corticosteroid drugs because they tend to deplete this mineral from your body. Small doses of corticosteroids rarely trigger problems, but as your dosage and length of treatment increase, so does the risk of side effects. While taking these drugs, limit your salt, and add more apricots and other potassium-rich foods to your diet.

2 **Pick a date for more potassium.** This sweet treat is near the top of the list of foods that can top off your potassium supply. A single deglet noor date — the most common eating variety — has more than 50 milligrams of potassium. Eat dates plain, or seeded and stuffed with fillings such as almonds, candied citrus peels, or marzipan. You can also chop them up and use them in puddings, bread, cakes, and other desserts.

Watch out!

Gluten and lectins may make your rheumatoid arthritis (RA) worse. Both are found in grains like wheat, oats, barley, and rye. There is no scientific proof, but a gluten-free diet has been known to improve RA symptoms. Lectin plant proteins may spur your immune system to attack your joints and cause RA. Not everyone has these allergies, but if you have RA, you might want to look into it.

3 **Slice a cup of strawberries.** You'll have an all-day dose of vitamin C, an important nutrient in the fight against arthritis. Your body needs vitamin C to make collagen, a key building block for the cartilage that protects your joints. Without vitamin C, those joints may weaken three times faster. As nature's leading antioxidant, vitamin C also fights against damage from free radicals all over your body. Plus it slows the development of osteoarthritis by keeping your tissues from aging as quickly. But don't be tempted to go overboard and take more than the daily recommended 90 mg for men and 75 mg for women. Another study found that osteoarthritis was worse in guinea pigs that took high doses of vitamin C over a long period of time.

New!

Pumpkin seed oil has a strong nutty flavor and is prized by chefs as a "culinary discovery." It may also ease the aches of arthritis. It has a store of omega-3 fatty acids, selenium, vitamin E, beta carotene, and other antioxidants that can all help get your joints moving. Find this unique treat in health and gourmet food stores or through the mail, and use it in salad dressings or for regular cooking.

4 **Pick a papaya and save your knees.** Papayas are full of a little-known nutrient called beta cryptoxanthin, a powerful antioxidant that scientists think can hold back arthritis in your knees. Beta cryptoxanthin is a carotenoid that can be converted to vitamin A. Since rheumatoid sufferers tend to have too many free radicals and not enough antioxidants, experts think all antioxidants may help relieve, or even prevent, rheumatoid arthritis. Specific research with beta cryptoxanthin has shown it reduces the risk of both RA and OA. Papaya fruit can be yellow, orange, pink, or red, depending on the variety, and it tastes like a cross between melons and peaches. A small papaya has more than 1,100 micrograms of beta cryptoxanthin, plus more than 100 percent of your daily requirement for vitamin C.

5 **Substitute almonds for a copper bracelet.** Folklore says copper bracelets relieve arthritis symptoms. Scientists believe the anti-inflammatory features of this trace mineral help relieve pain and swelling and that the standard American diet is copper deficient. But you're better off getting copper from food instead of wearing it. Most doctors believe bracelets do little good, and you can get your entire 900-microgram daily recommended intake of copper from a 3-ounce handful of almonds. For best results, choose either dry-roasted or plain almonds. They have slightly more copper than those that are honey-roasted or oil-roasted.

6 **Eat apples and ease arthritis stiffness.** Research suggests boron is essential to bone and joint health, and there is about a milligram of this important trace mineral in every pound of apples. Scientists believe 3 to 10 mg of boron a day could help prevent arthritis and also relieve morning stiffness and other arthritis symptoms. Most people only get 1 or 2 mg of boron a day, maybe because they eat more fast, processed food instead of fresh fruits and vegetables. So boost your body's boron by eating apples and dried fruit like raisins, dates, and prunes every day.

Learn more about the benefits of monounsaturated fats in the feature section *The truth about fat* on page 136.

7 **Switch to olive oil.** It has healthy monounsaturated fat, so it's an excellent substitute for butter or margarine. Scientists aren't sure if it's the monounsaturated fat or its strong antioxidant powers that helps olive oil stop inflammation in your joints. But research at the University of Pennsylvania has just uncovered another possibility for olive oil's pain-relieving power. It contains oleocanthal, a compound that seems to work much the same way as the nonsteroidal anti-inflammatory drug ibuprofen.

8 **Chew cherries when pain appears.** Long a folk remedy for gout, cherries now have scientific proof of their pain-prevention powers. Research at Michigan State University found the anthocyanins in cherries stop the enzymes that make prostaglandins, chemicals that cause inflammation and pain. The scientists say this delicious, vitamin-packed fruit relieves arthritis pain as well or better than aspirin, ibuprofen, and other nonsteroidal anti-inflammatory drugs. A bowl of 20 cherries a day during a bout with gout is enough to neutralize the aches and swelling, with no stomach upset or other side effects. The MSU study was done with laboratory tests, but a later study on people in California reported the same pain-relief results.

9 **Go after gout with wonderful water.** It's a double-barreled solution for this painful condition caused when crystals of uric

Kitchen TIP

Fresh tart cherries — the kind you use for pies and cobblers — will keep for 8-10 months if you freeze them. Place washed, stemmed, and pitted cherries on a cookie sheet so they don't touch each other. Freeze until they're solid, then transfer them to regular freezer bags.

acid form in your joints. Water helps dilute and flush the uric acid out of your body. It also lubricates and cushions your joints, much like a waterbed cushions your body, so it helps other arthritis as well as gout. Six to eight glasses of water a day is a good rule of thumb, but you may need more when you exercise. Johns Hopkins Medical Institutions say to drink enough to produce about two quarts of urine a day.

10 **Sip a cup (or two) of coffee.** A Japanese study found that men who drank a lot of coffee seemed to have less uric acid — the substance that causes gout — in their bodies. Green tea didn't affect uric acid, so the researchers believe it is something besides caffeine that makes the difference. Later research in Poland got the same result, especially among women who drank more coffee. Talk to your doctor before relying on coffee to cure your gout, though. Even though it's low in the purines that break down into uric acid, there is some concern that coffee's diuretic qualities might lower fluid levels and concentrate more uric acid in your body.

Duck a bout with gout

Food with high levels of purines can sometimes spark a gout attack. If you've had gout in the past, talk to your doctor about avoiding these high-purine foods.

- liver, kidneys, and other organ meats

- turkey, bacon, and veal

- gravy and consommé

- alcohol

- anchovies, sardines, herring, haddock, codfish, and trout

- mussels and scallops

11 **Get milk for gout.** A study published in the *New England*

Journal of Medicine confirms advice given as long ago as the 17th century — dairy products in your diet help get rid of gout. The study followed 47,000 men for 12 years and found that eating more low-fat dairy products along with less red meat and seafood significantly cut the risk of gout. Earlier research revealed that 30 grams of dairy protein a day — about four cups of milk — lowers blood levels of uric acid. If you're prone to this type of arthritis, a change in diet may be all it takes to soothe the problem.

12 **"Fish" for a better diet.** Protein and unsaturated fat, two key nutrients in fish, are critical parts of a different diet to do away with gout. Scientists think the 40-30-30 plan fights gout better than the old idea of simply cutting out many popular high-purine foods. The first part of the plan is to cut your calories to 1,600 a day. Next manage those calories so that 40 percent come from carbohydrates, 30 percent come from fat, and 30 percent from protein. Surprisingly, punching up your protein will help lower uric acid. Just make sure the fat that comes along with the protein is unsaturated. Eat more fish instead of red meat, and you'll get both protein and the right kind of fat.

A better way to rout gout

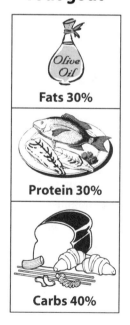

Fats 30%

Protein 30%

Carbs 40%

13 **Gobble garlic to rub out RA.** You're at greater risk for rheumatoid arthritis when your body's low on selenium and other antioxidants, and garlic has plenty of both. Selenium is an anti-inflammatory, and some experts believe it may reduce your swelling and pain. They also think any increase in antioxidants may relieve or even prevent RA. That's because rheumatoid sufferers tend to be low on antioxidants and overloaded with the free radicals that antioxidants wipe out. New research links low selenium with a higher risk of knee osteoarthritis, too. Selenium content often depends on the soil where a food was grown, but garlic is always generally high in this important mineral.

Skip the bottled tea

Eight out of 10 tea drinkers choose bottled iced tea rather than brewed tea. Unfortunately, the two beverages don't have equal health benefits. Dr. Jeffrey Blumberg of Tufts University points out that bottled tea is usually full of sugar and very weak, which means it has a lower dose of antioxidants. Its phytonutrients are also light sensitive, so they disappear after sitting in a clear bottle for a few days.

14 **Enjoy a cup of tea.** Tea is full of antioxidants and other anti-inflammatory agents. Research says tea and other antioxidant-rich fare may help fend off rheumatoid arthritis and relieve its symptoms. You can brew tea from the roots and leaves of all sorts of plants, but true tea — green, black and oolong tea — comes only from the *Camellia sinensis* plant. Of the true teas, green tea is generally recognized as the most healthful. Ginger tea is an herbal tea that can also ease inflammation and aches because ginger contains curcumin, an antioxidant with pain-fighting powers.

15

"Beef" up your inflammation fighters. Scientists searching for the next big thing in weight loss may have found an answer to arthritis pain instead. A polyunsaturated fatty acid called conjugated linoleic acid (CLA) — marketed as "the fat that fights fat" — may also cut down on pain in your joints. Cartilage cells inflamed by osteoarthritis produce chemicals that send pain messages to your brain, which make your joints hurt. Based on laboratory studies, researchers at Texas Tech and Penn State universities think CLA can keep these message-sending chemicals in check. Tests on humans are needed to know for sure, so take it easy with CLA supplements, and look for food sources instead. CLA is found in meats like beef and lamb and dairy foods like milk and cheese.

Cure aches with brown rice

In China the word for rice is also the word for food, but Chinese rice folklore goes beyond simple cuisine. An ancient Chinese cure for aching bones involves mixing toasted brown rice with minced ginger root and simmering them in liquor. This is combined into a cloth compress and rubbed on the painful joint.

16

Keep canned salmon on hand. You'll be less likely to be bothered by arthritis. It's full of vitamin D, which helps you absorb calcium from foods and keep the right amount of calcium in your blood. It also cuts your chances for osteoarthritis in your knees and hips, and seems to slow OA down if you've already got it. Additional research shows that older women who get more vitamin D have a lower risk of rheumatoid arthritis. As you get older, your skin loses its ability to convert sunlight into vitamin D. Cloudy weather and short winter days are also reasons to eat more food with vitamin D. Look no further than your pantry.

Just 3 ounces of canned sockeye salmon has more than your daily requirement of vitamin D no matter what your age.

17 Block OA with pomegranate juice. A study published in 2005 reveals that extracts from this ancient fruit can upset the development of osteoarthritis. A protein molecule called interleukin-1b promotes enzymes that cause OA cartilage to break down. Pomegranate juice seems to slow down the work of these enzymes. Prior to this study, scientists discovered that pomegranates have strong antioxidant and anti-inflammatory powers for a variety of other diseases. The discovery that it can stop the deterioration of human cartilage is especially important because current treatments for OA don't do much to slow it down.

TIP
Serving

The pomegranate has hundreds of tiny juice sacs held together by a leathery skin. The trick is to separate the tasty juice from the rest of the fruit, which is tough and bitter. An easy way is to cut the fruit into pieces and put them into a bowl of water, then scoop the tiny sacs out with your fingers. When you're done, remove the skin, strain out the water, and enjoy the luscious fruit that's left.

18 Add wheat germ to your breakfast. It has extra vitamin E, a powerful antioxidant that may ease joint inflammation and slow down the progress of osteoarthritis. The risk of rheumatoid arthritis increases when you're low on vitamin E as well. Heating destroys vitamin E so you don't reap its benefits if you eat a lot of fried or highly processed foods. When you sprinkle wheat germ on your breakfast cereal, you get an even bigger boost because many cereals are fortified with vitamin E. You can also mix wheat germ into pancake, waffle, and muffin batter; biscuits and bread; and meatloaf and other homemade foods.

19 **Fix an Indian dish like curry.** It's a great way to get curcumin — a phytochemical that reduces inflammation — into your diet. Curcumin is the active ingredient in turmeric, an important spice in Asian cooking and the key to curry powder, found in practically every Indian dish. Turmeric has been used as a medicine for centuries, and curcumin is a proven antioxidant. However, it's turmeric's anti-inflammatory power that's important if you have arthritis. Many herbalists say it gives relief from pain and swelling as well as ibuprofen and other NSAIDs, but without side effects. The Arthritis Foundation thinks turmeric may even be powerful enough to fight the stiffness and swelling of arthritis.

Foods that aggravate OA

Sometimes the food you eat aggravates your arthritis. If you suspect a certain food is touching off extra pain and swelling, stop eating it until you get better — then eat it again and see if the aches come back. Here are some foods that may make osteoarthritis worse.

▸ milk and other dairy products

▸ wheat

▸ shrimp

▸ certain red meats and poultry

▸ nightshade plants such as tomatoes, potatoes, bell peppers, and eggplant

▸ oranges

▸ peanuts

A Closer Look
Inflammation gone haywire

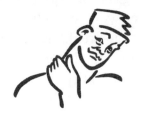

It sounds like a plot for a science-fiction movie. Something within you, something your body needs, suddenly turns against you — leading to chaos and death. Cue creepy music.

Only it's not a movie. It's all too real. Your body really features a necessary process that can go haywire. It's called inflammation, and it has been linked to everything from arthritis to Alzheimer's disease (*see box*).

Good guy gone bad

Ideally, inflammation acts as a hero. It is your immune system's normal quick response to a threat, such as an infection or injury. White blood cells rush to the scene of the crime and release chemicals to fight the intruder. The resulting inflammation restores order and protects you. But sometimes these powerful immune cells overdo it, sort of like swatting a fly with a hammer. Then the inflammation — marked by redness, heat, swelling, and pain — becomes a bigger problem than the original threat.

Your immune system can also run amok and unleash its inflammatory chemicals on normal tissue. That's what happens in autoimmune disorders like rheumatoid arthritis. When you have arthritis, you know about inflammation all too well. But not all inflammation has noticeable symptoms. Blood tests can detect elevated levels of the chemicals — such as C-reactive protein, interleukin-6, tumor necrosis factor-alpha, and fibrinogen — involved in your immune system's inflammatory response.

Secret source of health problems

In general, the suffix "-itis" — as in gastritis, bursitis, or tonsilitis — refers to inflammation of that particular body part. So it's easy to tell inflammation is involved in those conditions. But sometimes inflammation works behind the scenes — and what you don't know may hurt you. Just because you don't notice inflammation doesn't mean it's not causing trouble.

Here are just a few of the health conditions to which inflammation has been linked.

▸ **Arthritis.** Misdirected inflammation leads to some forms of arthritis, such as rheumatoid arthritis and gout.

▸ **Heart attack and stroke.** It's not just "clogged" arteries anymore. Experts now believe inflammation plays a major role in these events. In fact, higher levels of C-reactive protein mean a higher risk for heart attack and stroke.

▸ **Cancer.** Inflammation may interfere with normal cell death and produce DNA-damaging free radicals, leading to cancer. Normal inflammatory processes may even help the cancer spread.

▸ **Macular degeneration.** Researchers recently discovered a gene that may increase your risk for this leading cause of blindness. The gene normally prevents inflammation from running amok in the retina, but a variation of the gene has the opposite effect. Blood levels of C-reactive protein are also high in those with macular degeneration.

▸ **Gastrointestinal problems.** Inflammatory bowel disease, which includes Crohn's disease and colitis, can wreak havoc with your whole digestive system. Even ulcers, once thought to be caused by stress or spicy foods, stem from inflammation triggered by a bacterial infection.

Scientists keep finding more evidence supporting inflammation's role in disease. Don't be surprised if you hear more about it.

Fight inflammation with food

The most common treatments for inflammation involve anti-inflammatory drugs, including statins, aspirin, and ibuprofen. But you can also reduce inflammation through your diet. So stop paying high prices for costly supplements. You can make meals that are packed full of natural joint rebuilding nutrients, such as omega-3 fatty acids and antioxidants. Try eating more fatty fish, fruits, and vegetables, and cooking with olive oil and natural anti-inflammatory spices like turmeric and ginger.

On the other hand, you also need to keep your fat intake low. High-fat meals can trigger inflammatory responses. Beware of trans fats, the processed fat found in hydrogenated oils. They, too, may trigger inflammation, particularly in people with heart problems, according to a recent study. Luckily, starting in 2006, manufacturers must list trans fats on food labels.

Amazing Alzheimer's link

Today's inflammation may be tomorrow's Alzheimer's disease, a recent study suggests.

Researchers studied pairs of Swedish twins in which only one twin had dementia. The twin with dementia was four times more likely to have had gum disease earlier in life. Gum disease is an indication of exposure to inflammation.

Preventing infectious diseases early in life may be a way to prevent Alzheimer's later.

Other studies have shown that aspirin and ibuprofen may help reduce the risk of Alzheimer's disease — more evidence that inflammation may be involved.

Bone builders

19 foods to help you stay strong

Bad bones bother more than 64 million Americans. As many as 44 million either have or are at risk for osteoporosis, and 20 million more suffer from osteoarthritis, which may destroy the cartilage surrounding the joints in your bones.

Bone is living, growing tissue made up of collagen and calcium. All during your life, new bone replaces old bone. When you're young, you build bone faster than you lose it, and your skeleton becomes larger, heavier, and stronger. At around age 30, resorption — bone loss — slowly begins to outpace formation — new bone growth.

When you lose bone too quickly or form it too slowly, your bones become porous (osteoporosis means "porous bones") and more likely to break. Women in the first few years after menopause are hit hardest by this condition, but it also affects men.

A lifetime of low calcium means you set yourself up for low bone mass, rapid bone loss, and high fracture rates. But calcium also needs other nutrients — like vitamins C and D, potassium, and magnesium — to be effective. These nutrients are extremely important during your bone-building years. But they also help if you have already been diagnosed with osteoporosis.

The bottom line — good nutrition is a critical means to keeping your bones strong throughout your life.

1 **Keep bones growing with tomatoes.** Cells called osteoblasts constantly form new bone, while osteoclasts resorb or remove old bone. It's a constant process, and as you get older you begin to lose bone faster than you replace it. But the lycopene in tomatoes may help keep this cycle in your favor. Laboratory studies have found that lycopene seems to stimulate osteoblasts to grow better. This makes your bones stronger and helps you fight off osteoporosis. Tomatoes are the best-known source of lycopene, which is even stronger in tomato products like ketchup and tomato sauce. Many other nutrients in tomatoes — including vitamins A, C, and K, potassium, manganese, magnesium, and copper — are also important to good bone health.

New!

It's not just the calcium in milk that helps your bones. Exciting research from the University of Auckland in New Zealand reveals that lactoferrin — a glycoprotein found in milk — can stimulate bone-forming cells in the laboratory. Scientists think lactoferrin has potential for healing osteoporosis and regulating bone growth.

2 **Build up your calcium with powdered milk.** Calcium is the basic building block of good bones, and milk is the most familiar place to get it. But sometimes getting enough calcium can be a problem. One way to beef up your intake is to add nonfat dry milk to your diet. You can strengthen the milk you drink with it, or mix it in when you make breads, casseroles, and desserts. Since it's nonfat, it's an easy way to boost your calcium intake without the weight gain you get from many other dairy products.

3 **Boost bones with broccoli.** One of the few non-dairy foods full of calcium that your body can absorb easily, broccoli also has plenty of potassium and magnesium that make it possible for your bones to use the calcium. But vitamin C may be an even more important bone-boosting ingredient in broccoli. Your body needs vitamin C to build collagen — a fiber that holds bones, teeth, and cartilage together. Experts say vitamin C seems to slow the damage of osteoporosis and may even help repair damaged cartilage. Only peppers and certain fruits and fruit juices have more vitamin C than broccoli.

4 **Cook cauliflower instead.** If broccoli isn't your bag, cauliflower is another collagen-building crucifer. Like it's green cousins, these white flowerets are also excellent sources of vitamin C. In addition to low saturated fat, very low cholesterol, and lots of dietary fiber, both vegetables also have vitamin K, another important element for bone health.

Watch out!

Too much vitamin K combined with warfarin — an ingredient in many blood-thinning drugs — can cause dangerous blood clots. If you take those drugs, be careful how much vitamin K you get. Normal intake of foods with vitamin K shouldn't be a problem, but don't take supplements or go on a broccoli binge without your doctor's approval.

5 **Develop D with fortified milk.** Without vitamin D — the sunshine vitamin — your digestive tract can't absorb calcium from the foods you eat. When calcium doesn't come in, your body takes what it needs out of your bones, and that weakens your skeleton and causes osteoporosis. Normally, your skin converts sunlight into the vitamin D you need. But sometimes circumstances — like cloudy weather — prevent this process. That's when you need to get your supply from somewhere else. Most milk has vitamin D added to it, which makes it easy to get both your calcium and the nutrients it needs to keep your bones strong.

6 **Fill up on apricots.** Bones are not built on calcium alone. They need help from potassium and magnesium to make use of the calcium. Scientists know fruits and vegetables with these important minerals make a big difference in stronger, denser bones. Delicious dried apricots make a healthful snack and are a good source of potassium. Just a cupful of these tiny treats has almost a third of your daily requirement of potassium, plus a bonus of about 10 percent of the magnesium and 6 percent of the calcium you need. Add those dried apricots to a cup of trail mix for even more of these minerals — especially the magnesium.

7 **Find magnesium in bananas.** It's the most popular fruit in the United States and is often described as an ideal food. And although potassium may be its best-known nutrient, the banana also supplies a healthy dose of magnesium. Both minerals are needed for your body to absorb the calcium necessary for strong bones. Tests have shown calcium levels in your body will rise when you take in the proper amount of magnesium, even if you don't get extra calcium from food or supplements.

8 **Pick a perfect pineapple.** Eat a cup of fresh pineapple, and you've just given your body almost 80 percent of the manganese it needs for the day. This trace mineral is necessary for building bones and connective tissue. If that's not enough, pineapple is also full of vitamin C, which you need to make collagen — a fiber that holds bones, teeth, and cartilage together. Vitamin C also helps keep calcium in your skeleton instead of being reabsorbed into your blood. Canned pineapple and pineapple juice are also good sources of manganese and vitamin C, but watch out for added sugar.

9 **Fix baked beans for supper.** Other trace minerals are also important to bone building. One study found that postmenopausal women who were given supplements that included copper, manganese, and zinc lost less bone mass

Non-dairy foods with calcium		
Food	**Amount**	**Calcium (Mg)**
Total raisin bran	1 cup	1,000
Collards, frozen, cooked	1 cup	357
Sardines, canned with bone	3 oz	325
Blackeyed peas, fresh	1 cup	211
Pork and beans, canned	1 cup	149
Okra, fresh	1 cup	123
Almonds, raw	1 oz	70
Broccoli, cooked	1 cup	62
Oranges, raw	1 orange	52

than those who received no supplements. A good way to get zinc is to open up a can of baked beans — or make them from scratch. Along with zinc, you'll get a nice dose of copper, potassium, and magnesium, plus calcium. Check the table for other non-dairy foods that are good sources of calcium.

10 **Bolster your bones with barley.** You may not think of barley as often as you do other cereals, but it's the world's fourth-largest grain crop. It has all the whole-grain healthiness of wheat, rice, and corn — especially trace minerals like copper, which helps form collagen, a protein that is an important part of bones and connective tissue. The fiber in barley also helps protect the cells that build up your bones because of its ability to lower cholesterol. Research has found that high cholesterol is associated with fewer bone-forming cells in your body. An extra benefit of barley is that the entire kernel contains fiber, unlike many other grains where fiber is found only in the outer bran layer.

Beware of calcium robbers

Some foods you eat may take away the calcium you need for your bones. That's because of a natural compound called oxalate, which combines with calcium and keeps your body from using it. Foods high in oxalates include:

▸ spinach

▸ rhubarb

▸ beet leaves

▸ nuts

▸ chocolate

▸ strawberries

11 **Fortify calcium with the iron in grits.** Once a woman passes menopause, her recommended daily allowance for iron drops from 18 mg per day to 8 mg. However, scientists have discovered that keeping up your iron level also keeps up your bones. A study of post-menopausal women found that those who took in around 18 mg of iron and between 800 and 1,200 mg of calcium a day had better bone mineral density than those who got more or less of either mineral. Iron supplements without a doctor's advice can be dangerous, so eat iron-rich foods like fortified hot and cold cereals. For a change-of-pace breakfast treat, try grits. One packet of instant corn grits has your base RDA of 8 mg iron. Look on the label to make sure, though. Not all varieties of grits have the added iron you need.

12 **Spread on peanut butter.** Boron is involved in the metabolism of calcium and other minerals, and it may help estrogen stop osteoclasts from breaking down your bones. Most people get 1 or 2 mg of boron a day, but experts believe 3 to 10 mg a day may be better. It takes more than nine apples or about a pound and a half of peanuts to get 10 mg of boron, but you can still get a boron boost by putting peanut butter on apple slices for between-meal snacks.

13 **Drink tea for strong bones.** Fluoride in tea is just as good for your bones as it is for your teeth. Tea also has certain flavonoids that increase bone density as well as extracts that help calcium stay in your bones. You don't have to drink a lot of tea, just drink it regularly. Researchers in Taiwan compared tea-drinking habits and bone strength of more than a thousand Chinese men and women. They found that people who drank tea at least once a week for more than 10 years had better spine, hip, and total body bone strength than less frequent tea drinkers.

14 **Add onions to your diet.** They may help ward off osteoporosis and other bone-thinning diseases. Researchers at the University of Bern in Switzerland fed rats a fraction of an ounce of onion each day and found they were significantly less likely to lose bone. They believe a specific onion ingredient — gamma glutamyl peptide — slows down the activity of the osteoclasts that remove old bone. Unfortunately, you would have to eat almost a pound of onions a day to get the same dose the rats got. But these preliminary findings suggest it may be smart to make onions a regular part of your diet.

TIP
Serving

Tofu comes in a block that looks a lot like soft cheese. You can cut it up and use it in stir-fries, soups, or salad dressings. It has no taste so it takes the flavor of whatever you cook it with. Substitute tofu for meat, cheese, or yogurt, or just add a few cubes to any recipe for an extra healthy kick.

15 **Take tofu to avoid fractures.** Estrogen helps your body absorb calcium and kills off the osteoclasts that break down bone cells. So when menopause stops your estrogen supply, your bones are among the things that suffer. You lose bone at an increased rate for at least five years. One solution to this problem is tofu and other soy products. Their phytoestrogens and isoflavones provide dietary estrogen to make up for what your body no longer produces. It seems to work, too, according to recently published research. A sampling of 24,000 postmenopausal Chinese women over three years found significantly fewer bone fractures in those who ate the most soy protein versus the ones who ate the least. Just don't overdo it. Soy has been linked to other problems, such as senility and an increased risk of breast cancer.

16 **Choose cottage cheese for lunch.** It's a good source of vitamin B12, and a lack of this vitamin can lead to a broken hip, especially if you're an older woman. Several studies have linked either low B12 or high homocysteine to increased bone loss, particularly in the hips of women over 65. Vitamin B12 neutralizes homocysteine — a natural product of metabolism that weakens collagen and is also linked to heart disease and mental decline. A cup of cottage cheese contains about half your daily requirement of vitamin B12.

17 **Crunch carrots to score an A.** Recent research reveals you're also more at risk for hip fractures if you get either too little or too much vitamin A. So how do you get just the right amount of this important vitamin? Eat carrots, sweet potatoes, and other foods that contain beta carotene, a substance your body converts to vitamin A. Retinol, the active form of A, is found in animal foods, fortified foods, and supplements. Excess retinol is stored in your body fat and liver and can reach toxic levels as well as promote weak bones. But with beta carotene, you only convert as much as you need to keep your eyes, skin, and bones in good shape.

18 **Help yourself to herring.** This tiny delicacy is one of the cold-water fishes rich in omega-3 fatty acids. Although both omega-3 and omega-6 fats are important to your nutrition, some people eat as much as 25 times more omega-6 than omega-3. Experts recommend a ratio of between 4 to 1 and 10 to 1. Recent research from the University of California now associates higher bone density with better omega-3 to omega-6 proportions, which you can get by eating more fatty fish and less meat, milk, and processed food. (*See table for examples.*) The most common form of herring is a young, immature fish that has been steamed, seasoned, smoked, and packed into a sardine can. Larger herring are filleted and sold as kippers.

Foods with mostly omega-6 fatty acids	Foods with mostly omega-3 fatty acids
Chicken, pork, beef, and other lean meat	Salmon, sardines, cod, and other cold-water fish
Oils: sunflower, safflower, corn, cottonseed, peanut	Oils: canola, flaxseed, fish
Milk and eggs	Green leafy vegetables
Processed and fast foods	—

19 **Pick prunes to prevent bone loss.** Dried plums — the fruit formerly known as prunes — are known for their antioxidant power, but research at Oklahoma State University has found they may also slow down osteoporosis after menopause. One study showed a positive effect on the bones of postmenopausal women who ate 12 dried plums a day for three months. A more recent animal study showed that dried plums actually helped restore bones after losses had occurred. More study is needed, but the researchers believe the phenolic and flavonoid compounds in prunes may make a big difference in fighting osteoporosis.

A Closer Look
Dodging dangerous drug interactions

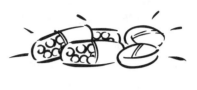

You wouldn't invite a Hatfield to the McCoy family reunion, wear a striped shirt with plaid pants, or put aluminum foil in the microwave. Some things just do not go well together.

That's especially true when it comes to medication. Some drugs should not be taken with certain foods, herbs, supplements, or other drugs. Not only may you lessen the effectiveness of the drug, you may also experience serious side effects.

Learn how to protect yourself with this handy guide to food-drug, herb-drug, and drug-drug interactions.

Food fiascos

To eat or not to eat? That is a key question when taking medicine. Some drugs work better when taken with food, while others work better on an empty stomach. For instance, you should take aceta-minophen on an empty stomach because food may slow its absorption. On the other hand, corticosteroids and nonsteroidal anti-inflammatory drugs (NSAIDs) should be taken with food or milk because they can irritate or upset your stomach.

Once you determine whether or not to take your pills at mealtime, you have to figure out what you can eat. Sometimes, food and drugs go together like peanut butter and jelly. Other times, it's more like oil and water. Here are some combinations to avoid.

▸ **MAO inhibitors and tyramine.** Foods containing the amino acid tyramine can cause a potentially fatal increase in blood pressure if you're taking these antidepressants. Avoid aged cheeses, processed meats, yeast extracts, soy sauce, beer, and red wine.

▸ **Blood thinners and vitamin K.** If you're taking blood-thinning drugs, like warfarin, limit your vitamin K. Found in spinach, broccoli, kale, turnip greens, brussels sprouts, and cauliflower, vitamin K promotes clotting and will lower the effectiveness of your medication.

▸ **Certain medications and grapefruit.** Grapefruit juice intensifies the effects of certain drugs, including statins, calcium channel blockers, blood pressure medication, and cyclosporine. Play it safe and avoid grapefruit when taking any medication.

▸ **Digoxin and oatmeal.** When eaten in large amounts, the fiber in oatmeal and other cereals may block the absorption of this heart medicine.

▸ **Tetracycline and calcium.** Foods containing calcium, such as milk or other dairy products, may reduce the absorption of this antibiotic.

▸ **Any medication and alcohol.** Alcohol blocks the effects of some medicines and dangerously increases the effects of others. It can also boost your risk for side effects, including nausea, vomiting, abdominal cramps, and headache.

Caffeine may also have an effect on your medication. Avoid mixing caffeine and bronchodilators, anti-anxiety drugs, histamine blockers, and some antibiotics.

Herb horrors

It's not just food you have to worry about. Herbs and dietary supplements may seem safe because they're "natural," but they can still interact with your medication. Watch out for the following herb-drug pairings.

▸ **St. John's wort and antidepressants.** Instead of feeling twice as good, you'll get a double dose of trouble. This combination can trigger what is called a serotonin syndrome. You may become confused, hot, sweaty, and restless, and experience headaches, stomachaches, muscle spasms, or seizures.

St. John's wort also weakens the power of several other prescription drugs, including digoxin, warfarin, cyclosporine, antibiotics, sedatives, birth control pills, cholesterol-lowering drugs, anti-psychotics, theophylline, and protease inhibitors.

▸ **Garlic, ginkgo, vitamin E and blood-thinning drugs.** These natural blood-thinners keep your blood from clotting. When combined with blood-thinning drugs, like warfarin or aspirin, they could lead to dangerous internal bleeding. Papaya can have the same effect.

▸ **Yohimbine and tricyclic antidepressants.** This herb, used to overcome impotence, can boost your risk for high blood pressure when taken with some forms of antidepressants.

▸ **Ginseng and phenelzine.** Combining ginseng with this MAO inhibitor may lead to mania in depressed patients.

▸ **Oil supplements and NSAIDs.** In rare cases, fish oil, borage oil, and evening primrose oil could trigger bruising and nose-bleeds if taken with aspirin or other NSAIDs, such as ibuprofen or naproxen.

If you're scheduled for surgery, stop taking all supplements two to three weeks ahead of time. They can cause complications such as bleeding, heart instability, low blood sugar, and changes in blood pressure.

Drug disasters

When you take multiple medications, you multiply your risk of drug-drug interactions. Sometimes, taking two similar drugs can lead to big problems. For instance, you can experience excessive sedation and dizziness if you take a sleep aid along with another drug with sedative effects.

Conversely, you may take two drugs whose effects oppose each other. This could make one or both drugs less effective. Say you're taking diuretics and NSAIDs. Diuretics help your body get rid of excess salt and fluids, but NSAIDs cause salt fluid retention — and, hence, make the diuretic less effective.

At other times, one drug might change how your body absorbs, distributes, metabolizes, or excretes another drug.

Make sure to let your doctor know which medications — including herbs and supplements — you're taking so he can help you avoid any dangerous interactions. If you have more than one doctor, tell each of them everything you're taking.

Always read and follow all label instructions carefully, and check expiration dates on over-the-counter drugs. If you do have any side effects, contact your doctor or pharmacist right away.

Cholesterol blasters

19 foods to sweep your arteries clean

Cholesterol is not a total bad guy. You actually need this soft waxy substance to help form certain hormones, cell membranes, and bile. The problem is, unlike some nutrients, cholesterol cannot dissolve in your blood. It needs molecules called lipoproteins to carry it through the bloodstream. The two main types of lipoproteins are low-density lipoprotein (LDL) and high-density lipoprotein (HDL).

LDL is what gives cholesterol its bad name. It can build up on the walls of your arteries and form a hard deposit called plaque. This plaque narrows your arteries and makes it harder for your heart to pump blood through them. If a blood clot forms, it can block blood flow completely and cause a heart attack or stroke.

HDL cholesterol, on the other hand, travels away from your arteries to your liver. Eventually it's flushed out of your body. This "good" cholesterol actually protects you from heart disease and stroke.

By keeping your LDL and total cholesterol levels low and your HDL levels high, you have a better chance of avoiding heart disease. Research has shown that the foods you eat can make a difference.

1 **Grab a handful of almonds.** They are loaded with monounsaturated fat — a type of fat that lowers your cholesterol. It does this by slashing the LDL or "bad" cholesterol that clogs your arteries without harming the HDL or "good" cholesterol. People in one study who ate about 4

113

ounces of almonds each day saw their total cholesterol plummet by 20 points over nine weeks. In another study, people who added almonds to their diets lowered total cholesterol by 7 percent and LDL cholesterol by 10 percent.

2 **Roast chestnuts any time of the year.** These nuts have very little fat, but it's mostly monounsaturated, so they, too, help keep your arteries clear. Plus you get 4.3 grams of fiber in just 10 chestnuts, which goes a long way toward preventing cholesterol buildup.

TIP
Storing

Keep your apples fresh and crisp. Leave them in the refrigerator instead of in a bowl on the counter. A temperature of about 32 degrees is ideal. Protect apples that are already cut by placing them in a solution of one part citrus juice to three parts water. Do this and you can be sure your next apple pie will be a hit.

3 **Learn the art of eating artichokes.** Making these a regular part of your diet will boost your bile production — an important step in reducing cholesterol. Bile helps break down cholesterol from the fat you eat. But that's not all. Luteolin, a compound in the leaves, may prevent new cholesterol from forming in your liver. Just watch what you pair these delicacies with. Skip rich, buttery sauces, and choose a low-fat veggie dip. Try a light mayonnaise blended with lemon juice or plain yogurt mixed with Dijon mustard.

4 **Snack on apples.** They are full of pectin, a natural and safe ingredient that can lower cholesterol — up to 30 percent if you eat it every day. This soluble fiber binds with harmful LDL cholesterol, carrying it out of your body, thereby preventing your small intestine from absorbing extra fats. If you want to lower your cholesterol with soluble fiber, experts say you should get results by eating 6 to 40 grams of pectin every day. One delicious apple provides 1.5 grams.

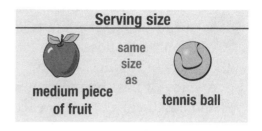

Serving size

medium piece of fruit — same size as — tennis ball

5 **Choose whole grains like barley.** Barley contains a form of soluble fiber called beta-glucan, which turns soft and sticky, slowing things down in your stomach and small intestine. This gives your body more time to whisk harmful cholesterol away so it can't gum up your arteries. Barley is a top-notch choice for boosting your daily fiber. See how it stacks up against three popular grains.

Grain (cooked)	Fiber in 1/2 cup
Pearled barley	3 grams
Long-grain brown rice	1.75 grams
Couscous	1.1 grams
Long-grain white rice	0.6 grams

6 **Serve black beans at your next potluck.** By eating beans instead of a fatty meat, you put a good dent in your daily dose of cholesterol. And they fill you up without lots of calories — only 225 calories in a one-cup serving. A study of healthy men showed that when they ate about two and a half cups of beans each day, they ate significantly less fat and reduced their total cholesterol levels. Black beans are a tasty addition to soups and salads, but others, like navy and kidney beans, work well, too.

7 **Prevent gallstones with peaches.** Gallstones are solid masses of cholesterol that form in the gallbladder or bile ducts. Lower your chances of these potentially painful stones by eating peaches. They contain vitamin E, a nutrient that helps prevent gallstones from developing. Peaches are also on a list of foods researchers found cause no pain in people with gallstones. Other friendly foods on the list include beef, rye, soy, rice, cherries, apricots, beets, and spinach.

Watch out!

Stay away from curry if you have a history of gallbladder problems.
Turmeric, the main ingredient in curry, can aggravate a gallstone or other blockage of the bile duct. The same goes for pure turmeric spice. Avoid it, as well, if you take a blood-thinning drug such as Coumadin, warfarin, or NSAIDs, or if you have bleeding problems. The curcumin in turmeric adds to the effect of these medicines.

8 **Sprinkle on the wheat germ.** Mix a little wheat germ into your next bowl of cereal or yogurt. A French study found that eating a quarter cup of raw wheat germ a day for 14 weeks lowered total cholesterol by 7.2 percent and "bad" LDL cholesterol by 15.4 percent. The secret ingredient may be vitamin E, which is known to prevent LDL cholesterol from oxidizing and turning into a sticky plaque in your arteries.

9 **Sneak in some flaxseed.** The seeds of the flax plant have tons of soluble fiber, a miracle fiber that helps protect against high cholesterol, high blood pressure, heart disease, and even obesity and cancer. Not only is it loaded with fiber, flaxseed is also one of the best sources of omega-3 fatty acids, a polyunsaturated fat that keeps your blood from sticking. Plus, it is a rich source of plant lignans, phytochemicals that act like antioxidants. All these potent cholesterol fighters explain why studies have shown flaxseed can lower this damaging fat by as much as 14.7 percent. Sneak ground flaxseed into oatmeal, rice pilaf, applesauce, or yogurt for an easy and healthful addition to your diet.

Add variety to your cooking

Flaxseed oil and olive oil are both popular for their flavor and cholesterol-lowering abilities, but they're not the only show in town. Try one of these cooking oils next time you want to whip something up and bring your cholesterol down.

▸ sesame oil

▸ peanut oil

▸ canola oil

▸ soybean oil

▸ walnut oil

▸ almond oil

▸ grapeseed oil

10 **Spice things up with ginger.** Add flavor to your meals and help your arteries at the same time. This spice contains phytochemicals like gingerol and shogaol that fight atherosclerosis. A 1-inch chunk of fresh ginger every day can lower LDL cholesterol, reduce triglycerides, and prevent LDL oxidation. Studies show that ginger also prevents blood from clotting in your arteries. Look for it in your favorite Asian recipes.

11 **Cut up a clove of garlic.** It can cut down on fat buildup in your arteries by lowering LDL cholesterol and leaving your HDL cholesterol

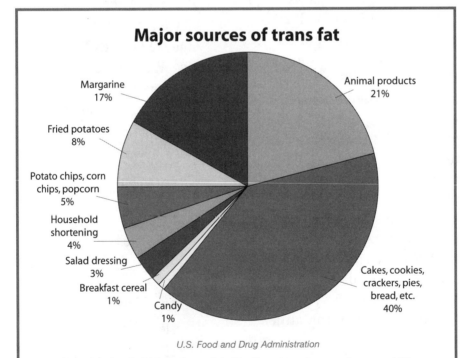

Major sources of trans fat

Margarine 17%

Animal products 21%

Fried potatoes 8%

Potato chips, corn chips, popcorn 5%

Household shortening 4%

Salad dressing 3%

Breakfast cereal 1%

Candy 1%

Cakes, cookies, crackers, pies, bread, etc. 40%

U.S. Food and Drug Administration

Avoid eating foods high in trans fat. Studies show it can raise your LDL cholesterol levels and increase your risk of coronary heart disease. The graph above shows major sources of trans fat for American adults. You can use it as a guideline or check nutrition labels on foods to find out how much trans fat they have.

unharmed. It also decreases triglycerides and improves circulation. Garlic's healing powers come from sulfur compounds like ajoenes, allicin, and allyl sulfides. Studies show these sulfur compounds work together to protect you from cholesterol buildup. Allicin is only released when garlic is crushed or chopped so take the time to prepare it properly. Let the crushed garlic sit for 10 minutes before cooking to give this powerful compound time to activate.

12 **Pour a glass of grape juice.** Drinking two glasses of purple grape juice a day is a natural way to rejuvenate your veins and arteries that will have you feeling brand new. This sweet beverage contains several ingredients that make it a heart-smart choice. Quercetin, a flavonoid found in grape skins, acts as an antioxidant to prevent LDL cholesterol from collecting on your artery walls. Resveratrol, also found in the skin, thwarts inflammation and blood clots. Meanwhile procyanidins in the seeds help keep blood vessels relaxed and exert antioxidant powers of their own. When these substances are combined, the mixture can reduce platelet clumping by 91 percent. Studies even show that one serving of grape juice is as good for your heart and arteries as a daily dose of baby aspirin. So drink up!

13 **Be creative with mushrooms.** This is one fungus you won't mind having around. Mushrooms are a good source of chromium, a mineral that acts as an antioxidant. Studies show chromium can help lower your LDL cholesterol while raising "good" HDL cholesterol levels. You can add fresh or sautéed mushrooms to soups, salads, spaghetti sauce, and countless other dishes.

14 **Sweeten the deal with honey.** A recent study found that eating honey might reduce cholesterol levels after just a couple of weeks. People who took a honey solution every day for 15 days experienced a 7 percent drop in LDL cholesterol and a 2 percent rise in good HDL cholesterol. Honey is a good source of dietary antioxidants, which may be the key. Sweeten your next cup of tea with a spoonful of honey, and savor the benefits.

New!

The old Mars bar you know and love just got a nutritional makeover. Mars has developed a chocolate bar with soy plant sterols, cocoa flavonols, added calcium, and B vitamins, all of which are good for your heart. The cocoa flavonols may help your arteries stay healthy by keeping LDL cholesterol from oxidizing and clogging them up. This new treat is part of the Mars CocoaVia brand of chocolate bars that you can find in most supermarkets. Good nutrition never tasted sweeter.

15 **Indulge in some chocolate.** This delectable treat has something to offer besides calories — mainly a generous helping of antioxidants called polyphenols. A 1.5-ounce piece of chocolate has as many polyphenols as a glass of red wine. These antioxidants can help your heart by keeping LDL cholesterol from becoming oxidized, which can harm your arteries. A study in Finland showed the polyphenols in dark chocolate may be even better because they also raise your good cholesterol levels. But don't go overboard. Like most things, chocolate is healthful only in moderation.

16 **Cook up some homemade tomato sauce.** You'll reap the benefits of lycopene, an antioxidant that keeps your arteries flowing free by breaking down cholesterol. Research has shown that the more lycopene you get, the lower your chances of clogged arteries. Processed tomato products like tomato sauce may give you more lycopene than raw ones. So get out your favorite recipe, and fill your home with the heavenly aroma of fresh tomato sauce.

17 **Fix a bowl of oatmeal.** Good, old-fashioned oatmeal does more than stick to your ribs. Oats have beta-glucan, a sticky kind of soluble fiber that helps slow the movement of food through your intestine. This gives HDL particles more time to pick up cholesterol and carry it away to your liver for disposal. A recent Canadian study of overweight women showed that eating two oat bran muffins a day for four weeks lowered their total cholesterol. The FDA recommends having four servings of foods with beta-glucan — a total of 3 grams — every day to lower your risk of cardiovascular disease. Oatmeal counts, and so does oat bran cereal.

18 **Catch a fish for dinner.** There are plenty of fish in the sea, but the fat ones are the best at lowering cholesterol. Fatty fish like tuna, mackerel,

Don't forget to read the label

Let's say you walk through the baked goods section of your grocery store and see an item you like. It's advertised to be reduced-fat and a good source of fiber. Will it help your cholesterol levels? Not necessarily. Look at the nutrition label. If it lists "partially hydrogenated oil" as an ingredient, then it has trans fats, and those can elevate your cholesterol.

and salmon are rich in omega-3 fatty acids, a polyunsaturated fat that can protect your arteries from damage. Omega-3 reduces triglycerides so they don't build up on artery walls. Then it thins your blood so it can flow better. You won't get that kind of action from lean fish like flounder and haddock.

New!

Yoplait Healthy Heart is a new low-fat yogurt with plant sterols. These are extracts from vegetable oil that help keep your small intestine from absorbing cholesterol. A study shows that eating two servings of Yoplait Healthy Heart yogurt every day for a month may reduce LDL cholesterol by an average of 6 percent. Benecol Spreads have a similar ingredient called plant stanol esters, which also block the absorption of cholesterol. Replace your usual butter or margarine with Benecol Spreads for a tasty way to lower cholesterol.

19 Dish out some yogurt. Ever since scientists linked fermented milk to the clear arteries and healthy hearts of the Maasai, a remote African tribe, they have been studying the cholesterol-lowering effects of yogurt. And most clinical studies have shown that yogurt may have a modest effect. One study that used a yogurt drink enriched with plant sterols found it brought down LDL cholesterol and total cholesterol. Scientists aren't sure why, but the key seems to be eating yogurt with live cultures on a daily basis.

A Closer Look
Get smart about your heart

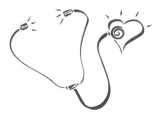

James Brown calls himself "the hardest-working man in show business." But the Godfather of Soul has nothing on your heart. Without missing a beat, your heart works non-stop to pump blood throughout your body. Quite simply, your heart keeps you alive. Alas, too often, its reward for a lifetime of hard work is neglect or abuse. That's why heart disease is the leading cause of death in the United States. Fortunately, through diet and lifestyle changes, you can lower your risk.

Breaking down heart disease

Several related conditions contribute to heart disease. Here is a brief description, including risk factors and symptoms, of some of the main ones.

Atherosclerosis. The narrowing and thickening of your blood vessels comes from the buildup of cholesterol-rich plaque. This blocks your blood flow, increasing your risk of stroke, heart attack — even death. Researchers now suspect inflammation plays a key role in the development and progression of atherosclerosis.

▸ People with high cholesterol, high blood pressure, and diabetes are at greater risk. Smoking, obesity, stress, and a lack of exercise also contribute.

▸ There are no early symptoms. Later signs include pain in the chest, arm, jaw, or back; heart attack; and stroke.

High blood pressure. Blood pressure is the force of your blood pushing against your arteries. You suffer from high blood pressure, or hypertension, when your heart must work harder than normal to pump blood through your circulatory system. This can damage both your heart and your arteries and boost your risk of heart attack, stroke, kidney failure, eye damage, congestive heart failure, and atherosclerosis.

▸ People over 60 and blacks are at greater risk. Being overweight and inactive, smoking, drinking, stress, and a diet high in salt and fat can also contribute.

▸ There are no visible symptoms. The main warning sign is a blood pressure reading higher than 140/90.

High cholesterol. Your body needs cholesterol to build cell walls and make hormones. But too much of this soft, waxy substance can be deadly. It builds up on your artery walls, causing blockages that lead to heart attack or stroke. Low-density lipoprotein (LDL) is called bad cholesterol because it carries cholesterol to your arteries. High-density lipoprotein (HDL) is the good guy that transports cholesterol to your liver, where it is eliminated.

▸ Overweight, inactive people, smokers, and those who eat lots of saturated fat get high cholesterol. Older people and diabetics are at greater risk, and family history also plays a role.

▸ There are no outward symptoms. Watch out for total cholesterol over 200 mg/dl, LDL levels over 130 mg/dl, and HDL levels under 40 mg/dl.

Stroke. A stroke, or "brain attack," damages your brain the way a heart attack damages your heart. Some strokes are caused by blood clots that block the flow of blood to the brain (ischemic stroke), while others happen when a blood vessel in the brain ruptures (hemorrhagic stroke). As with a heart attack, fast action can save your life.

▸ Two-thirds of all stroke victims are over 65 years old. Blacks are also at greater risk. Other risk factors include a personal or family history of stroke, high blood pressure, heart disease, and diabetes. Smoking and a lack of exercise are also major factors.

▸ Symptoms include numbness or weakness, especially on one side, confusion, trouble speaking or understanding, difficulty seeing, dizziness, loss of balance or coordination, and a sudden, severe headache.

How food can help

While the above conditions work together to damage your heart and blood vessels, eating the right foods can help keep your heart in tip-top shape. Often, the same food will provide protection from a variety of heart problems. As an added bonus, a heart-healthy diet also protects you from other diseases, like cancer or diabetes.

Make room for helpful foods such as fish, olive oil, fruits and vegetables, whole grains, nuts, seeds, and beans. Herbs and spices like garlic and ginger can help thin your blood and improve circulation, plus they make terrific alternatives to salt when seasoning your food.

At the same time, you want to limit saturated fat, found in meat and dairy products, and salt. Saturated fat boosts your cholesterol, while sodium can raise your blood pressure.

Lifestyle changes lower risk

You can't eliminate all your risk factors. For instance, you can't stop yourself from aging or change your family history. But you can do something about the others. Besides eating right, you can also take these simple steps to improve your lifestyle — and reduce your risk for heart disease.

- **Exercise.** Regular exercise not only keeps your weight in check, it also helps lower your blood pressure and LDL cholesterol. A brisk 30-minute walk each day will help.

- **Quit smoking.** This might be the most significant step you take to protect your heart.

- **Limit alcohol.** If you drink, do so in moderation. A good rule of thumb is no more than two drinks per day for a man and one for a woman.

- **Lose weight.** Being overweight boosts your risk of several heart-related conditions. A good diet and exercise program will help you maintain a healthy weight.

- **Relax.** Find ways to reduce stress, whether it's listening to soothing music, gardening, or just spending time with your family.

Even if you adopt a healthy diet and lifestyle, you may need prescription medication to control your blood pressure or cholesterol. Always follow instructions carefully.

Considering how hard your heart works for you, it's about time you did something for it. So, have a heart — and start taking the necessary precautions to save yours.

Heart disease by the numbers

Don't let heart disease sneak up on you. Make sure you know your blood pressure and cholesterol levels. Here are the numbers to remember.

Blood pressure		Cholesterol		
Under	Ideal	Under	Over	Ideal
140/90	120/80	200 Total	40 HDL	
		130 LDL		100 LDL

Heart smarts

17 foods to bring your blood pressure down

Your life may depend on your blood pressure. Hypertension — high blood pressure (HPB) — hits around 50 million people in the United States and a billion worldwide. It can trigger coronary heart disease, congestive heart failure, stroke, and kidney disease. HPB causes two-thirds of the strokes, almost half of all heart attacks, and is the biggest risk factor for death in the world.

Two key ways to control HPB are to lose weight and watch what you eat, but doctors sometimes prescribe medication for mild high blood pressure just because they know most people won't follow their diet and exercise advice. You might avoid those expensive little pills by simply adopting a healthy lifestyle.

Diets that keep blood pressure down are heavy on fruits, vegetables, whole grains, and fiber, and light on salt, red meat, saturated fat, and cholesterol. The minerals potassium, magnesium, and calcium are also important, as are vitamin C and omega-3 fatty acids.

1 **Bake with barley.** Or try eating it plain, or serve it in soups and casseroles. It's one of the best grains you can eat for blood pressure control. Not only does barley have more fiber than any other grain, it also contains potassium and magnesium — two of the top minerals for fighting high blood pressure. Pearl barley — the most common barley product — has been polished to remove the hard outer

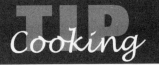

TIP
Cooking

Barley flour has more than three times the fiber of wheat flour, but it doesn't have the kind of gluten to make baked goods rise properly. For best results, mix it with regular wheat flour. For yeast breads, substitute barley flour for about a quarter of your total flour. For cookies and quick breads, use half and half.

shell. It can be served as a side dish in place of rice or pasta or as an extra ingredient in many kinds of recipes.

2 **Try a stalk of celery.** It's an old Asian remedy for high blood pressure. Modern scientists think phthalides — the chemicals that give celery its unique taste and smell — also reduce cholesterol and relax the smooth muscles that line blood vessels to ease your blood pressure. Even if it doesn't have a magic ingredient, celery is loaded with other blood pressure friendly nutrients. Fiber, folate, potassium, and vitamin C are just a few of celery's selling points. It does, however, have more sodium than many other vegetables, so don't go overboard. As with all foods, eat celery in moderation, and cut back on salt somewhere else.

3 **Score another victory for broccoli.** This glorious green vegetable seems to be good for everything, and your blood pressure is no exception. Broccoli sends at least four important fighters into the battle against high blood pressure — calcium, potassium, magnesium, and vitamin C. Countless studies show that people with low levels of these nutrients tend to have raised blood pressure. Calcium and potassium help your body get rid of sodium through your urine. Potassium and magnesium relax blood vessels and improve blood flow. Vitamin C is an antioxidant that also strengthens your blood vessels. Get the most out of your broccoli by steaming it or eating it raw. Water-soluble nutrients like vitamin C are lost when you boil it or microwave it in water.

4 **Nibble on dried apricots.** They make a great snack, and they give you iron, potassium, magnesium, beta carotene and copper — high-voltage nutrients that help control blood pressure and prevent heart disease. The potassium alone in apricots does wonders for your heart. It protects your blood vessels from damage, prevents dangerous irregular heartbeats, and keeps your blood pressure down. If you like fresh fruit better than the dried kind, look for fresh apricots from California and Washington on your grocer's shelves during June, July, and August.

5 **Eat the whole beet.** People from ancient Greece to Renaissance Italy only ate the green beet leaves and threw away the red roots. But it was still a smart move because just a half cup of beet greens gives you more potassium than a medium banana. Potassium is even more important for your blood pressure if you take diuretics to keep it low. These medicines remove this mineral from your body along with water. Eating red beets still gives you some potassium, but you also get a good dose of folate, a B vitamin important in neutralizing homocysteine and warding off heart attacks and strokes. So buy the whole beet, greens included, and find ways to use it all in your cooking.

6 **Spin magnesium magic from spinach.** Magnesium is just one of several key nutrients in spinach, but it may be called a miracle mineral since researchers have found so many health conditions it guards against. It protects your heart, lowers your cholesterol, fights cancer, and much more — from avoiding diabetes to preventing migraine headaches. At age 70, you absorb only about 65 percent of the magnesium you did at age 30, so it's important to eat plenty of spinach and other magnesium-rich food, like whole grains, beans, avocados, nuts and seafood.

Chocolate — a boon to blood pressure?

Chocoholics may have even more reason to rejoice. A recent Italian study suggests dark chocolate may lower blood pressure. The secret is the flavonoids that abound in dark chocolate. The study control group ate white chocolate, which lacks flavonoids, and they saw no improvement. Milk chocolate, which most people favor, only has low amounts. To be sure you reap the benefits of this luscious treat, switch to the dark variety.

7 **Season with garlic and onions.** It's a good way to cut back on the salt that is so dangerous for your blood pressure. But garlic and onions do more than just add flavor to your food. Sulfur compounds in both these members of the allium family fight poor circulation by keeping blood platelets from clumping together and making your blood sticky. Quercetin and other flavonoids in onions also help stop LDL cholesterol from oxidizing and blocking your arteries. So spice up your meals with these flavorful additions to your menu. And watch out when eating packaged or restaurant foods. Experts recommend no more than 2,400 mg of sodium per day, and some, like those in the following table, may be packed with it.

Food	Amount	Sodium (mg)
Swanson's Hungry Man XXL Roasted Carved Turkey	1 pkg	5,410
Oscar Mayer Lunchables Deluxe Turkey & Ham w/Swiss & Cheddar	1 pkg	1,940
Stouffer's Slow Roasted Beef & Gravy Homestyle Dinner	1 dinner	1,510
Banquet Macaroni & Cheese Dinner	1 dinner	1,500
La Choy soy sauce	1 tablespoon	1,260
Cheese Fries w/ranch dressing	–	4,890
Reuben sandwich	–	3,270
General Tso's chicken w/rice	–	3,150
Spaghetti w/sausage	–	2,440

8 **Go for guava juice.** What you drink can affect your blood pressure just as much as what you eat. Juice is a good way to get the goodness of guava, because once it's ripe, the fruit itself only lasts a couple of days. Guava is a delicious tropical fruit that is packed with potassium and more than twice the vitamin C of an orange. Potassium helps your heart beat steadily, and vitamin C keeps your small blood vessels healthy. Research shows this winning combination can lower blood pressure several points.

9 **Snack on sunflower seeds.** They're loaded with vitamin E, a powerful antioxidant that stops LDL cholesterol — the bad kind — before it can form plaque that clogs up your arteries. It has other anti-clotting powers, too, so it's easier for your heart to pump blood and keep your blood pressure down. Vitamin E also guards against hardening of the arteries, stroke, and heart attack. Remove the tasty sunflower morsel from its shell, or buy the little seeds already shelled to sprinkle on salads or munch by the handful.

10 **Peel a banana.** Here is another fabulous fruit for a healthy heart. Potassium is one of the banana's most talked-about qualities, but that's not all it has going for you. Bananas also boast a couple of B vitamins — folate and vitamin B6 — that help you get rid of homocysteine, a normal byproduct of protein metabolism. When your homocysteine levels are high, you're at risk for heart disease, stroke, and clogged arteries. A balanced diet with lots of fruits, vegetables, and B vitamins keeps homocysteine from getting out of hand. Both potassium and folate help your blood vessels dilate, too, which lets more blood and oxygen get through and keeps your blood pressure low. Bananas are low in salt and fat and high in fiber and vitamin C, which make them an important part of a heart-healthy diet.

11 **Spread your bread with peanut butter.** It's a better choice than cream cheese, margarine/dairy butter, or fatty lunchmeat. Peanut butter has monounsaturated fat instead of the saturated fat found in other spreads, which is guaranteed to push up your blood pressure. Dietary Approaches to Stop Hypertension (DASH) diet and Mediterranean diet guidelines both emphasize monounsaturated instead of saturated fats. So put peanut butter — preferably the natural version — on your bagel, or fix a peanut butter sandwich instead of using meat. You'll find monounsaturated fat fills you up better, too, so you're less likely to overeat.

12 **Start out with oatmeal.** Just two servings of high-fiber cereal a day — one for breakfast and one later in the day — changed the diets of men in a recent study enough to meet the American Heart Association's recommendations for fat and cholesterol. The fiber was so filling that they automatically ate fewer fatty foods. Study after study proves that whole grains and dietary fiber lower your blood pressure and your risk for heart disease. Oatmeal is an excellent source of whole-grain goodness, and you can have it as a breakfast cereal or mix it into muffins, meatloaf, or other baked goods.

DASH drops blood pressure

One of the best plans for healthy blood pressure is the Dietary Approaches to Stop Hypertension (DASH) diet sponsored by the National Heart, Lung, and Blood Institute. It is proven to dramatically lower your blood pressure without additional risky drugs and consists of 10 simple steps — four don'ts and six do's. Don't go overboard with salt, fat, red meat, and sweet food and drinks. Do eat more fruit, vegetables, whole grains, low-fat dairy products, poultry, and lean fish.

13 **"Fish" for fewer BP problems.** Fish can help you lower your blood pressure in two ways — by enjoying the sport itself or by enjoying a fish dinner. Fishing is a good way to relax and drop your blood pressure, and eating your catch — providing it's a cold-water fish like salmon or mackerel — gets more omega-3 fatty acids into your system, which also brings down your pressure. Omega-3s help relax blood vessels and make your blood less sticky so it flows easier. They also help regulate your heartbeat and clean your artery walls of cholesterol and triglyceride fats. The American Heart Association recommends you eat fish at least twice a week because of its fatty acids and because fish is a good source of protein without the high saturated fat of meat products.

14 **Add flaxseed for more omega-3.** Flax has been used for thousands of years, both for eating and for making linen. Flaxseed oil has more omega-3 fatty acids than anything except fish, and the seeds are loaded with soluble fiber. You can bake with flax flour, or stir in flaxseeds to make crunchy cookies, breads, and muffins. Use the oil in salad dressings, soups, sauces, and baked goods. Just make sure you store it in the refrigerator so it stays fresh.

15 **Taste some tofu.** Recent studies have shown that soy protein may help bring down your blood pressure. Tofu is a form of soy protein that is easy to add to your diet. Substitute it occasionally for meat, cheese, or other protein-rich food. You should aim for 15 to 25 grams

Watch out!

Taking soy isoflavone supplements is not the same as eating tofu now and then. In at least one case, large doses of this supplement — used to relieve symptoms of menopause — caused a drastic rise in blood pressure. Soy isoflavones have also been linked to other health problems. Always ask your doctor before taking supplements instead of getting your nutrients from food.

of soy protein per day — the amount in one half to a cup of tofu. The jury is still out on whether more than that can increase your risk of other forms of ill health, including brain aging and memory loss.

16 **Benefit from a new nutrient in potatoes.** British researchers were recently surprised to find that potatoes contain kukoamines, a little-studied group of chemicals that lower blood pressure. They were previously known to exist only in a certain species of Chinese medicinal plants. Add this exciting new information to the fact that potatoes have always been a great source of fiber, vitamins C and B6, and potassium, and you have an excellent package of blood pressure protection. Potatoes have very little cholesterol, sodium, or saturated fat to begin with, but you have to be careful what you add to them. They are healthiest when boiled, baked, or mashed. The salt and fat that comes with fried potatoes and French fries will raise your blood pressure instead of lowering it.

17 **Heat up with chili peppers.** New research says hot foods may help keep away heart attacks. Scientists think cayenne and other chilies can slow blood clotting and even dissolve existing clots. Capsaicin, which gives chili peppers their heat, can help lower blood pressure, and researchers think it may also help lower cholesterol in your blood. So if you enjoy food that makes your eyes water, pop in another jalapeno. It may send your temperature up, but there is a good chance it will also bring your blood pressure down.

A Closer Look
The truth about fat

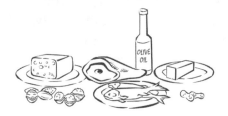

It's spelled f-a-t, but for many people "fat" is a four-letter word. Dieters and health-conscious eaters avoid it like the plague. That's because eating too much fat may contribute to obesity, heart disease, high blood pressure, cancer, diabetes, and other diseases.

However, your body needs some fat to stay healthy. Fats provide the raw materials for making hormones and bile. Other fats carry the fat-soluble vitamins — A, D, E, and K — in your bloodstream throughout your body. Fats also add to the enjoyment of eating by making food tender, tasty, and pleasant-smelling.

Fat's many forms

All dietary fats pack 9 calories per gram, as opposed to 4 calories per gram for protein or carbohydrates. But that doesn't mean all fats are created equal. Here's a look at the main types of fat.

Saturated fat. These fats, found mainly in animal sources like meat, milk, butter, and cheese, raise your cholesterol levels. While cholesterol in your blood can come from dietary sources of cholesterol, such as egg yolks, it mainly comes from saturated fat — which is also found in coconut, coconut oil, and palm oil.

Monounsaturated fat. This healthy fat lowers LDL cholesterol, the bad kind that clogs your arteries, and boosts HDL cholesterol, the good kind that whisks cholesterol to your liver and out of your bloodstream. Olive oil is a great source of monounsaturated fat, which can also be found in canola oil, avocados, and nuts.

Polyunsaturated fat. Like monounsaturated fat, these fats lower LDL cholesterol. However, they also lower HDL. There are two main types of polyunsaturated fat, called essential fatty acids.

▸ Omega-3 fatty acids, found mostly in fish, boast a wealth of health benefits. They not only reduce your risk of heart attack and stroke, they also help with arthritis, Alzheimer's disease, diabetes, cancer, and depression. You'll find omega-3 in fatty fish like salmon, tuna, mackerel, herring, and sardines. You can also find some in wheat germ, walnuts, flaxseed, and dark green leafy vegetables.

▸ Omega-6 fatty acids, found in vegetable oils like soybean, corn, safflower, and sunflower oils, are a key part of your diet. But too much omega-6 and not enough omega-3 can lead to headaches, arthritis, asthma, arrhythmia, and more.

Trans fat. This sneaky fat is a polyunsaturated fat gone awry. During processing, manufacturers turn some of a food's unsaturated fat into saturated fat to extend shelf life or change the taste or texture of that food. Trans fatty acids are one of the byproducts. This unusual kind of super fat raises your cholesterol as well as your risk for heart disease and possibly cancer. It shows up in hydrogenated vegetable oils and margarines.

Fat-tastic tips

Fat should not make up more than 30 percent of your total calories, and no more than 10 percent should come from saturated fat. Here are some more fat guidelines.

▸ **Cut back on saturated fat and trans fat.** Choose low-fat or fat-free dairy products and lean cuts of meat. Limit fast foods, bakery goods, chips, crackers, and mayonnaise.

▸ **Strive for a healthy ratio of omega-6 to omega-3.** Eat more fish, ditch deep-fried foods, and replace corn or soybean oil with canola or olive oil.

▸ **Read food labels.** As of 2006, you'll find trans fats listed under saturated fats.

▸ **Don't be fooled by low-fat or fat-free cookies.** That includes other snacks as well. Often, they just have more sugar and calories.

▸ **Keep some fat in your diet.** A recent study found that you don't absorb carotenoids, including beta carotene and lycopene, when you eat salad with fat-free dressing.

Below is a look at some common oils and their mixtures of fatty acids.

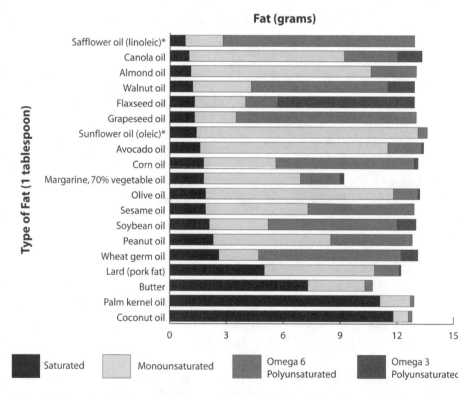

Fat (grams)

Some oils can be high in either monounsaturated (oleic) or polyunsaturated (linoleic) fats.

Source: USDA Nutrient Database for Standard Reference (Release 18)

Stroke straight talk

18 foods to safeguard your heart

Every minute, someone has a stroke. That's when a blood vessel becomes blocked (an ischemic stroke) or bursts (a hemorrhagic stroke), cutting off blood flow to part of your brain. Without oxygen in your blood, your brain cells die — and never come back. Depending on which part of your brain is affected, you could be paralyzed on one side of your body, lose feeling, balance, bladder control, or sight, or have trouble swallowing, talking, or remembering things. That is, if you survive.

Because of the serious damage it can do, stroke sometimes goes by a more serious name — brain attack. It's the third leading cause of death in developed countries, ranked behind only heart disease and cancer.

It so happens that heart disease and stroke are caused by the same thing – atherosclerosis. It occurs when cholesterol, fat, and other substances in your blood build up in the walls of your arteries and clog or block them completely. The process can begin when you're a child, but it may not become a problem until you're in your 50s or 60s. The good news is that changing your diet can prevent both of these dangerous diseases.

1 **Add walnuts to your diet.** You don't have to suffer a heart attack or stroke. Walnuts can thin your blood and help prevent clots. A study of 20 men and women showed that eating 8 to 13 walnuts a day can improve blood flow by making your arteries more elastic. Walnuts are rich in alpha-linolenic acid and gamma-tocopherol, nutrients that are known to be heart healthy. Researchers from Pennsylvania State University found that eating an ounce or more of nuts five times a week may bring down your risk of heart disease by up to 39 percent. When you're looking for a quick snack, a handful of nuts is the perfect choice.

2 **Consider an entrée of salmon.** This fish can help you live longer and keep your brain sharp. The omega-3 fatty acids in salmon fight forgetfulness, high blood pressure, weak bones, poor digestion, and even some cancers. Just two servings a week is all it takes to bolster your body against heart attack, stroke, diabetes, and depression. In a study of more than 2,000 men, researchers found that eating fatty fish like salmon on a regular basis may protect you from heart disease. Omega-3 fatty acids work by lowering blood pressure, making blood less sticky, and regulating your heartbeat.

Watch out!

Choose wild salmon over farmed salmon. Studies show farmed salmon typically have higher levels of contaminants like polychlorinated biphenyls (PCBs) than wild salmon. If you can, choose wild Alaskan salmon. Canned salmon is another option since it's usually cheaper and almost always contains wild Alaskan salmon.

3 **Peel open an orange.** One extra serving a day of this mouth-watering fruit can reduce strokes, lower obesity, and fight heart disease. Studies have shown a daily serving of citrus fruit can bring down your risk of stroke by nearly 20 percent. The magic ingredients — vitamin C, carotenoids, and flavonoids — all protect your heart from cardiovascular disease. The potassium, folate, and phytonutrients in oranges offer protection as well. As a bonus, eating fruit on a regular basis can help you avoid weight gain. A 12-year study of thousands of women revealed that the ones who ate the most fruit were less likely to become obese during middle age. Now that's a sweet deal.

4 Protect yourself with asparagus.

It is a delicious way to get folate, an important B vitamin. Just four spears of asparagus supplies you with 89 micrograms of folate — more than 20 percent of the 400 micrograms you need each day. Here's how it may help. High levels of a chemical called homocysteine in your blood can damage and narrow your arteries. That can increase your risk of heart disease, blood clots, heart attacks, and strokes. Scientists have long thought certain B vitamins like folate and B6 can lower heart disease risk by lowering homocysteine levels in the blood. A recent study has disputed this, however. *(See box)* To get some B6 and B12 with your folate, have a side of asparagus with a main portion of fish or turkey. This meal rich in B vitamins could be a tasty way to help your heart.

Do B vitamins protect against stroke?

A recent study from Norway contradicted the long-held belief that B vitamins help lower your risk of heart disease through their interaction with homocysteine. The study tracked volunteers taking B vitamin supplements for three and a half years. Although their homocysteine levels went down, their risk of heart disease did not. Instead, the ones who took both folate and B6 actually experienced a higher risk. Research is sure to continue, but in the meantime, avoid taking high doses of B vitamins without talking to your doctor first.

Pay attention to symptoms

Ischemic strokes are often foreshadowed by one or more "mini-strokes" that may only last a few minutes. Researchers have found these mini-strokes tend to come within a week of the major stroke. So get medical attention immediately if you experience any of these symptoms, no matter how minor.

▶ sudden change in vision

▶ sudden difficulty with speech

▶ unexplained or unusually severe headaches or dizziness

▶ sudden change in mental abilities

▶ impaired judgment

▶ sudden numbness, weakness, tingling sensations

▶ sudden change in personality

▶ any other symptoms, like paralysis, that happen on only one side of the body

5 **Take avocados to heart.** You'll have less heart disease, lower blood pressure, and less congestion from cholesterol. You might not expect a fruit that's second only to olives in fat content to be so good for cardio care. But its fats actually have properties that make them work for your benefit and reduce bad cholesterol levels. Add to that potassium and magnesium, vitamins C and E, and folic acid. These nutrients have proven to be more than a match for cholesterol, sodium, and homocysteine, all of which harm arteries and increase your chances of heart attack and stroke.

6 **Add cauliflower to your menu.** Research has found that the risk of ischemic stroke is 31 percent lower in people who eat more than five servings of fruits and vegetables a day, compared with people who eat less than three servings a day. Make sure one of those servings is cauliflower. Cruciferous vegetables like cauliflower seem to offer the most protection against stroke.

7 **Strike out strokes with bananas.** They are loaded with potassium. Just one medium piece of fruit has well over 400 milligrams, which is about 10 percent of your daily requirement. Potassium helps control blood pressure and is one of your most valuable weapons against stroke. You may cut your risk for these deadly "brain attacks" by up to 40 percent just by getting enough each day. Eat bananas — along with fruit juices, potatoes, tomato sauce, and beans — for the potassium you need to keep high blood pressure and strokes away.

8 **Beat heart disease with blueberries.** They protect arteries from free-radical attack and keep them open and strong. If left unchecked, free radicals scar your arteries, allowing them to be clogged by fatty deposits. The longer this goes on, the higher your risk for heart attack and stroke. That's where the antioxidant protection of blueberries comes in. Since blueberries are second only to red beans in terms of total antioxidant levels, you can put blueberries to work on your heart's behalf. It's certain you won't find a more delicious way to protect your heart anywhere.

9 **Remember to include brussels sprouts.** When you think of good sources of vitamin C, oranges and other fruits come to mind. But they don't have the market cornered. Brussels sprouts are also rich in this powerful antioxidant. *(See table)* Vitamin C neutralizes free radicals so they don't cause plaque buildup on your artery walls. This vitamin also keeps inflammation down. That explains why a study in Finland found that people who have a higher intake of vitamin C are 24 percent less likely to suffer from heart disease than those who don't get as much of the vitamin. Researchers in Belgium also found a link between low levels of vitamin C and certain types of atherosclerosis. Brussels

sprouts have a rather strong flavor, so try steaming them
until they're tender — roughly 10 to 15 minutes. Or stir-fry
them in olive oil and garlic for extra heart protection.

Source	Vitamin C
Sweet red pepper, 1 medium	226 mg
Papaya, 1 medium	188 mg
Cranberry juice cocktail, 1 cup	107 mg
Broccoli, 1 cup cooked	101 mg
Strawberries, 1 cup	98 mg
Brussels sprouts, 1 cup cooked	97 mg
Green pepper, 1 medium	96 mg
Orange juice, 1 cup chilled	82 mg
Kiwi fruit, 1 medium	71 mg
Orange, 1 medium	70 mg

10 **Steam brown rice for breakfast.** Lace it with cinnamon and raisins, and you'll have a much healthier meal compared to the standard bacon-and-egg fare. In a long-term study of more than 40,000 men, researchers found the men who ate the most fiber cut their risk of a fatal heart attack in half. And most of these men ate cereal for breakfast — a good start. You can cook brown rice the regular way — or set the timer on a rice cooker so it's waiting for you when you roll out of bed.

11 **Chew on a carrot.** You'll get a healthy dose of potassium and vitamin C — two ingredients that protect against heart disease and even boost your immune system. Vitamin C in particular strengthens your capillaries and lowers your risk of angina. Carrots also have their share of fiber. Studies show that people who get 25 to 40 grams of fiber a day may cut their risk of heart disease by 30 percent. Chop up a carrot to put in a stew or salad for a dash of color and heart protection.

12 **Mix it up with cranberries.** They aren't just for the holidays any more. The antioxidants, flavonoids, and polyphenols in cranberries can help protect you from heart disease. Researchers at the University of Wisconsin gave cranberry juice powder to animals with atherosclerosis for six months, and it helped blood flow by relaxing their blood vessels. Get the benefits and tart taste by sprinkling dried cranberries over a bowl of oatmeal, barley, or other cereal.

13 **Appreciate olive oil in a new way.** Experts have known for a while that olive oil is good for your heart. Its monounsaturated fats make your blood less likely to clot, which reduces your risk of stroke. But scientists have recently discovered a new compound in olive oil called oleocanthal — a chemical similar to ibuprofen. Not only does oleocanthal have the same pungent sensation in the throat as ibuprofen, it also has the same ability to reduce inflammation — an important step in preventing stroke and heart disease. Now you have another reason to pour on the "Italian butter." Try all the different types to find out which one is your favorite.

Type of oil	Flavor	Use
Virgin olive oil	Mild, fruity flavor	All-purpose cooking oil
Extra virgin olive oil	Robust, fruity flavor	Drizzle over salads or vegetables
Extra light olive oil	Mild flavor	Can replace vegetable oils

14 **Brew a pot of green tea.** You may want to think twice about your next cup of coffee and brew some green tea instead. A Harvard Medical School study found that tea drinkers had a lower risk of heart attack than java lovers. Scientists think theanine — an amino acid in green tea — makes blood less sticky so it can move smoothly through your arteries. Another study in the Netherlands found that older men who consumed the most fruits, vegetables, and tea were the least likely to die from heart disease or stroke. So relax your mind — and your arteries — with a cup of green tea.

15 **Feast on figs.** The triple punch of fiber, potassium, and magnesium in figs means extra protection from stroke, especially if you have high blood pressure. Experts agree that more nutrient-rich fruits and vegetables should be your first line of defense. Dried figs are especially good for you because they're chock-full of antioxidants. They also make a sweet and portable snack. For a different kind of dessert, dip fresh figs in vanilla or lemon yogurt. It will satisfy your taste buds and your heart at the same time.

16 **Try bulgur for a change.** Try a side of bulgur pilaf instead of potatoes and you'll add more than variety to your diet. Research shows eating whole grains like bulgur can reduce your risk of stroke. This delicious and healthy grain is made from wheat berries or kernels that have been steamed, dried, and cracked. It's sort of like cracked wheat except it's been pre-cooked. It has a hearty, nutty flavor and is easy to cook. And with all its insoluble fiber, protein, magnesium, iron, manganese, and B vitamins, bulgur will make a nutritious substitute for refined grains like white rice and bread that don't offer the same benefits.

17 **Be sure to eat your spinach.** This leafy vegetable is a good source of folate and magnesium — two nutrients that work to protect you from heart disease. A recent study out of Sweden showed that folate might protect against hemorrhagic stroke, although it did not show the same effect for ischemic stroke. Getting more than 450 milligrams of magnesium, another valuable nutrient, may bring down

TIP *Storing*

When it comes to storing spinach, colder is better. A recent study showed that fresh spinach stored at 39 degrees Fahrenheit — about the same temperature as a refrigerator — retained its nutrients longer. Spinach stored at 68 degrees — closer to room temperature — lost half its folate in four days. The same amount of nutrients disappeared in six days from spinach stored at 50 degrees. The spinach in the fridge didn't lose that much until after eight days. So keep your spinach refrigerated to reap the most benefit.

your risk of stroke by one-third. Just one cup of spinach supplies you with more than a third of that amount. It's easy to find ways to slip spinach into your diet. Add spinach leaves to your sandwich instead of lettuce, or mix them into your tossed salad.

18 **Pour yourself some pomegranate juice.** Researchers at the University of California recently found that pomegranate juice improves blood flow in people with ischemic coronary heart disease. Volunteers drank pomegranate juice every day for three months, and their blood flow to the heart improved by 17 percent. Try mixing the juice with club soda or sparkling water for a tasty and refreshing drink.

A Closer Look
Carbohydrates — friend or foe?

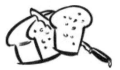

Just as your car needs fuel, so does your body. That's where carbohydrates come in. Carbohydrates — starches, sugars, and fibers that come mainly from plants — represent your body's main source of energy. They also help your brain and nervous system operate at peak performance.

Yet, to many dieters, "carbs" have become the enemy. But you don't have to give up carbohydrates to lose weight and improve your health — you just have to know how to choose the right ones.

Complex is best

Carbohydrates come in two basic forms — complex and simple. Here is a brief look at both of them.

▸ **Complex.** Your body needs these important starches and fibers. You get them from grains, breads, pasta, and vegetables, like white or sweet potatoes, corn, and dried beans.

▸ **Simple.** These carbohydrates, which are sugars, give you quick energy. Milk, fruits, and juices contain simple carbohydrates. They bring nutrients, like water, vitamins, minerals, and sometimes fiber, to your table.

Refined sugar, found in sugar, candy, desserts, and your sugar bowl, is also a simple carbohydrate. But it doesn't have any nutrients — just a lot of empty calories.

Carbohydrates should account for 45 to 65 percent of your total calories. Like protein, carbohydrates provide 4 calories per gram.

So that comes out to between 225 grams and 325 grams of carbs each day for a 2,000-calorie diet.

Most of these should be complex carbohydrates. For maximum health benefits, choose whole grains, which not only contain complex carbohydrates but also fiber and other important nutrients. Many of your favorite foods now come in whole-grain versions. You can even find whole-grain white bread.

Lowdown on low-carb diets

But what about all those people losing weight by following the Atkins Diet or other low-carb diets? These diets appeal to people because they let you load up on steak, butter, bacon, eggs, and other usual dieting outlaws. You cut carbohydrates without restricting fat or protein. Of course, as with any diet, you're also cutting down on your calories.

They also work — at least in the short term. Studies show some people lose more weight on this diet than on a low-fat diet. And surprisingly, studies also show this eating plan can lower cholesterol and improve blood sugar levels.

But remember, your diet must provide all the nutrients you need. When you limit vegetables, fruits, and grains, you put your health at risk. With all that meat comes a lot of saturated fat, which may increase your risk for heart disease, stroke, and cancer. The long-term health effects of these diets remain unknown.

Also, low-carb diets are often boring and hard to stick to. Once you go back to eating a normal amount of carbohydrates, your weight comes back, too. Not surprisingly, these diets have been waning in popularity. Rather than declare war on carbs, just make the right ones part of a healthy diet.

Sugar control

22 foods to help you triumph over diabetes

It may seem like diabetes is all about what you can't eat. In fact, fighting it has just as much to do with what you should eat as what you shouldn't.

Food and nutrients actually help your body regulate blood sugar and make the most of insulin. Certain compounds in food can even work like insulin in your body. What you eat can improve your insulin sensitivity, balance blood sugar spikes, and help prevent as well as treat diabetes.

Sometimes battling this disease is a matter of making smart food choices, like munching almonds instead of potato chips, or making pancakes with buckwheat flour instead of white flour. Other times, it's about adding specific foods to your diet, such as cherries.

Whether you are worried about developing diabetes or need help managing it now, there's a food to help you.

1 **Beat diabetes with bulgur.** Large studies have consistently shown people eating at least three servings of whole grains a day have a 20 to 30 percent lower risk of type 2 diabetes than people who eat only three servings a week. Now evidence suggests high-fiber whole grains like bulgur may also help prevent metabolic syndrome, a risk factor for both type 2 diabetes and heart disease. Fiber probably contributes to these protective benefits, but experts say there is more to it than that. Fiber from refined grains doesn't offer as much benefit as that from whole-grain foods. Scientists suspect

Feast on fiber

The American Diabetes Association recommends getting at least 35 grams of fiber each day, but a recent study found eating 50 grams of fiber daily helped diabetics keep blood sugar, insulin, and cholesterol all under control. A cup of cooked bulgur gets you well on your way toward reaching these goals with 8.2 grams of fiber. Besides that, it boasts loads of chromium, a mineral that makes insulin more effective.

whole grains slow down the digestion of other foods and limit how much sugar your body absorbs from carbohydrates. Whole, unrefined grains also pack more nutrients, particularly magnesium, a mineral that helps diabetics control blood sugar. So whether you're trying to prevent or manage this disease, you can bet on bulgur.

2 **Drive away disease with broccoli.** This little green veggie loads you up with magnesium, a mineral crucial to both preventing and controlling diabetes. Magnesium improves insulin sensitivity, and several studies show people who get the most magnesium from their diets lower their diabetes risk. Diabetics tend to be deficient in this mineral, especially if they take insulin. Evidence suggests boosting magnesium intake may help diabetics control blood sugar and protect against serious complications such as high blood pressure, heart, and vision problems. Your best bets for more magnesium — shop for fresh and organically grown foods. Processing removes this precious mineral, and experts say organic produce contains much more magnesium than conventionally grown vegetables.

3 **Splash on vinegar.** Honey may help you catch more flies, but vinegar chases off disease. This acidic juice seems to slow down the digestion of food, evening out

blood sugar spikes after a meal. In a recent study, people who were insulin-resistant — a condition that can lead to diabetes — drank a mixture of apple cider vinegar and water before eating. They saw their after-meal blood sugar drop 34 percent compared to those who drank a placebo, and they experienced smaller spikes in insulin and glucose. Evidence suggests just three teaspoons of vinegar can lower your after-meal blood sugar as much as 30 percent, while adding only two calories — and lots of flavor — to any meal.

4 **Wake up and smell the coffee.** A morning cup of joe could help prevent type 2 diabetes. Long-term studies show people who drink four or more cups of coffee every day lower their risk of developing the disease at least 28 percent. The real hero might not be caffeine at all but chlorogenic acid, an ingredient in coffee that helps regulate blood sugar. Coffee's high levels of antioxidants, mostly in the form of chlorogenic acid, may also improve insulin sensitivity by protecting your cells from damage. Other ingredients, including magnesium, potassium, and niacin, could also play key roles in staving off diabetes. In the short term, though, coffee actually raises your blood sugar, so people who don't normally drink it should not start just to prevent diabetes. For the same reason, some experts warn diabetics to avoid coffee.

5 **Go "fish" for more omega-3.** Obesity is a major risk factor for type 2 diabetes, so you might expect countries with high rates of obesity to have high rates of diabetes, too. That's true in places where people eat very little fish and seafood. But in countries where fish is common, extra weight does not increase the risk of diabetes. In fact, these fat, fish-loving countries have about the same diabetes risk as people in "skinny" countries. One study found eating 6 ounces (about two servings) of fish each week protected seniors from developing glucose intolerance. Thank the polyunsaturated "healthy" fat omega-3 for these amazing benefits. Experts say omega-3-rich foods like fish may cancel out some of the negative effects of being overweight. A diet rich in it seems to help cells release insulin and boost the action of insulin in your body.

Some foods seem to raise your risk of type 2 diabetes. Limit them to dodge this dangerous disease.

Instead of	Eat
red meat, hot dogs, bacon, sausage	poultry, fish
white bread	bread made from "stoneground" flour
refined white flour	buckwheat flour
highly processed foods	fresh whole legumes, fruits, and vegetables
sugary drinks like sodas	low-fat milk, water

6 **Ditch diabetes with dairy products like milk.** Out of more than 40,000 men studied for 12 years, men who got the most dairy every day were the least likely to develop type 2 diabetes, 23 percent less likely than men who got the least. What's more, for every extra daily dairy serving the men ate, their diabetes risk dropped another 9 percent. Experts suspect the calcium and magnesium in dairy foods might lower diabetes risk, while lactose and dairy protein could make people feel full longer, cutting back on the obesity that often leads to diabetes. But don't go diving into the ice cream yet. Chowing down on high-fat dairy foods like sour cream, whole milk, cream cheese, and other cheeses did not drop the men's risk. Only low-fat dairy products — including skim and low-fat milk, yogurt, sherbet, cottage cheese, and ricotta cheese — seemed to protect them.

7 **Beat high blood sugar with blueberries.** Sprinkling blueberries on your morning cereal could help control glucose. They've long been a favorite folk remedy for high blood sugar, and scientists may finally have found proof. Blueberries lowered blood sugar levels about 26 percent in animal studies. Grab a handful of these healthy berries for a tasty breakfast topping, energy-boosting smoothie, or sweet, simple snack.

8 **Battle disease with brussels sprouts.** Your cells produce renegade molecules known as free radicals as a natural part of normal body processes. Typically, you get enough vitamin C and other antioxidants from food to neutralize free radicals and keep them in check. But experts suspect this antioxidant defense mechanism stops working in diabetics, allowing free radicals to get out of hand. These rogue molecules damage cells and systems over time, leading to some of the serious vascular complications, like heart disease, that often develop in diabetics. Japanese researchers found people with diabetes have lower levels of vitamin C in their immune cells than healthy people, and that diabetics with complications had even less C than those without. You can fight back by eating more brussels sprouts and other high-C foods such as citrus fruits, strawberries, and broccoli. Besides putting the brakes on free radical damage, this vitamin can help control blood sugar levels and improve your insulin sensitivity.

9 **Add a dash of cinnamon.** The active ingredient in cinnamon, a polyphenol compound called methylhydroxy chalcone polymer (MHCP) mimics the action of insulin in your body. Insulin helps control blood sugar levels, but it also plays a part regulating triglyceride and cholesterol levels. That may explain why diabetics tend to have higher cholesterol and triglycerides in addition to higher blood sugar than most people. Cinnamon appears to lower blood sugar along with LDL cholesterol and triglycerides. Diabetics also tend to have high amounts of free radicals circulating in their bodies. Lab experiments showed cinnamon effectively neutralized these damaging molecules. What's more, a little dab may do it. People in studies benefited from taking just 1 gram — about half a teaspoon — of cinnamon each day.

> ### TIP
> ## Cooking
>
> Sprinkle cinnamon on oatmeal, cereal, toast, yogurt, apples, and other fruit; spice up cooked carrots, squash, sweet potatoes, and meats; or stir hot drinks with cinnamon sticks instead of a spoon. Don't eat cinnamon oil, though, which is poisonous even in small amounts.

10 **Get healthy as a horse on oats.** Oats contain a special form of soluble fiber known as beta-glucan. It's sticky, and it slows down the movement of food through your digestive tract so your body absorbs glucose more slowly and gradually. That's good news for diabetics, who need to keep tight control of blood sugar levels. Experts say doubling, even tripling, the amount of soluble fiber in your diet can improve glycemic control in people with diabetes. Oats can help you do that. Research has shown adding oat bran to meals lowers after-meal spikes in glucose and insulin better than wheat bran in both healthy people and those with type 2 diabetes. The form of oat you eat also plays a part — the less processed the grain, the better. Oats makes a great binder in recipes. Add one-fourth cup of oats to pancake batter or to meat loaves and patties.

11 **Lunch on lentils.** Building more beans, peas, lentils, and other legumes into your diet can help lower blood sugar as well as improve insulin sensitivity and glycemic control. But how you cook those legumes may be just as important as how many servings you eat. Processing and milling legumes and grains breaks down the walls between individual plant cells, making it easier for your body to digest and absorb the starch in those cells. That puts sugar in your blood stream faster, leading to blood sugar spikes

Food	Fiber content (grams)
Lentils, boiled (1 cup)	15.6
Black beans, boiled (1 cup)	15.0
Lima beans, boiled (1 cup)	13.2
Asian pear (1 large)	9.9
Boiled artichoke (1 cup)	9.1
Fresh raspberries (1 cup)	8.0
Dried plums (1 cup)	7.7
Fresh blackberries (1 cup)	7.6
Cooked squash (1 cup)	5.7

after meals. Eating whole beans and grains may prevent that spike, because they break down more slowly. In fact, your body may not digest these unprocessed foods completely, so some of the sugar may never make it into your system. Plus, unrefined legumes make you feel full longer than their processed counterparts, so eating the whole beans could help you lose weight.

A high-fiber diet can help you overcome insulin resistance, but cereals and whole grains aren't the only sources of fiber. Add variety with fiber-filled fruits, vegetables, and legumes like ones on the previous page.

12 **Toast some almonds.** Popping almonds may help ditch diabetes, thanks to monounsaturated fats (MUFAs). The American Diabetes Association (ADA) says MUFAs could help manage your insulin and blood sugar levels and fight diabetes-related heart disease. In fact, these special fatty acids make up a big part of the ADA's eating plan. Diabetics should aim to get 60 to 70 percent of their daily calories from a combination of carbohydrates and MUFA-packed foods, like almonds.

13 **Pick poultry for healthy protein.** Moderate amounts of protein may help balance your blood sugar. Unlike most refined carbohydrates, protein does not cause glucose levels to spike, making it a smart choice at mealtime. Most experts advise diabetics to get 10 to 20 percent of their daily calories from protein, and a new Finnish study suggests poultry may be the best way to do that. Out of more than 4,000 men and women, those who made poultry part of a healthy diet had less chance of developing type 2 diabetes. Just remember, moderate amounts of protein may benefit your blood sugar health, but experts warn against extreme high-protein diets for people with diabetes. Such a diet may affect how well your kidneys work and impact long-term heart health, both special dangers for diabetics.

14 **Spread on peanut butter for sugar control.** The little-known B vitamin biotin could do big things for managing diabetes. It helps your body use glucose and digest fats and carbohydrates, and it may even reduce the amount of insulin your body needs. A biotin deficiency keeps your body from using glucose properly, and studies have shown type 2 diabetics tend to have lower biotin levels than non-diabetic people. Animal studies found upping biotin intake increased insulin secretion, which would help lower blood sugar levels. You can get plenty of this vitamin naturally from the foods you eat, including peanut butter, cereals, legumes, and nuts.

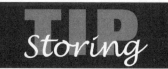

TIP
Storing

Use fresh artichokes within a few days, or sprinkle a few drops of water on them to keep them looking and tasting fresh for up to two weeks. Store them in an airtight plastic bag in your refrigerator.

15 **Eat artichokes to cut glucose.** This green giant may manage diabetes by helping your liver regulate blood glucose levels. The liver stores extra glucose in the form of glycogen, then turns it back into glucose when blood supplies run low. Some people have livers cranking out glucose their blood doesn't need. Animal studies show artichokes keep the liver from producing too much of this sugar, good news for people with type 2 diabetes.

16 **Sip on soy milk.** Soy protein may help prevent both kidney disease and coronary heart disease in people with type 2 diabetes. Fourteen men with kidney disease and type 2 diabetes added a soy protein supplement to their diet for two months. The supplement boosted kidney function, raised "good" HDL cholesterol, and improved the ratio of HDL to "bad" LDL cholesterol. Soy contains isoflavones, compounds that act like the hormone estrogen. Experts say estrogen may slow down the progression of kidney disease. Soy products can be helpful if you are lactose intolerant or have wheat sensitivities. You can substitute one cup of soy flour plus one-fourth cup potato starch in place of one cup wheat flour in recipes.

17 **Serve up shellfish.** Many diabetics suffer from moderate zinc deficiency. If you're one of them, you may have trouble keeping your blood sugar level normal after a meal. A zinc shortage could also contribute to vision problems down the line, such as retinal damage and loss of night vision. An occasional serving of shellfish can keep you swimming in this mineral. Women over the age of 50 need 8 milligrams (mg) of zinc daily, while men over 50 should shoot for 11 mg a day. Just 3 ounces of Alaskan king crab dishes out about 6.5 mg of zinc. Steam oysters, crab, or other shellfish in season for a flavorful change of pace. Allergic to seafood? Bulgur, oat bran, lentils, and chickpeas all pack plenty of zinc, too.

18 **Get tempted by apples.** Chromium helps your blood deliver and use insulin, guarding your body against insulin resistance and hypoglycemia. In test after test, scientists found that people who get more chromium have greater control over their blood sugar levels and are less likely to suffer from diabetes. Apples provide plenty of this important mineral, but you must eat the skin, too. These tempting fruits are also full of soluble fiber, which helps slow down the release of glucose into the bloodstream. Try dipping apple slices in low-fat or all-natural peanut butter for a burst of biotin, too.

19 **Pick cherries to prevent diabetes.** Looking for a sweet way to beat diabetes? Start with cherries. In a new lab study, researchers at Michigan State University put some mice on a high-fat diet and others on a low-fat diet. The high-fat mice quickly gained weight, developed fatty livers, and became glucose intolerant. Researchers then began feeding them anthocyanins, compounds found in cherries, in addition to their fatty food. After eight weeks, these obese, glucose-intolerant mice had lost weight, lowered their cholesterol, raised their insulin levels, were more glucose-sensitive, and once again had healthy livers. The researchers used Cornelian cherries but say the more popular tart cherries are similar.

Watch the sugar

Dried fruits make great snacks, but they tend to have more sugar than their fresh counterparts. Take this into account when trying to get more fruit in your diet. Otherwise, dried and fresh fruits are nutritionally the same.

20 **Balance blood sugar with buckwheat.** This grain may help lower blood sugar levels after meals, thanks to a compound known as D-chiro-inositol (D-CI). Canadian researchers gave buckwheat extract or a placebo to rats with type 1 diabetes after eating. Within two hours, the buckwheat rats had almost 20 percent lower blood sugar than those on placebo. In a separate study, eating biscuits made from buckwheat flower lowered blood sugar in diabetics. Make a pasta salad or stir fry with soba noo-dles, a Japanese pasta made from buckwheat. Or make a stack of flapjacks using buckwheat flour instead of white. It won't cure diabetes, but it could offer a cheap, simple, safe way to control blood sugar and cut the risk of heart, kidney, and nerve damage from diabetes.

Act fast to treat low blood sugar

Diabetics who use insulin sometimes take too much, resulting in low blood sugar (hypoglycemia). Over-the-counter glucose tablets and gels are probably the best treatment for hypo-glycemia because they contain pure glucose, so they reach your blood stream faster. Don't try treating low blood sugar with foods like chocolate or nuts. These contain fats, which slows their diges-tion. Stick with these choices instead:

▸ two to five glucose tablets

▸ 4 ounces orange juice

▸ 6 ounces non-diet soda

▸ five to seven hard can-dies

21 **Go ga-ga for guava.** The Chinese have used the guava fruit to treat diabetes for many years, and now experts know it may lower blood sugar. Research also shows guava helps lower blood pressure, reduce LDL choles-terol, raise "good" HDL cholesterol, and even protect against heart disease. Hard to believe one humble fruit can do all that. Plus, it's loaded with good-for-you nutrients, includ-ing beta carotene, lycopene, potassium, and soluble fiber — and it packs more than twice as much vitamin C as an orange. Grab a guava and get on the bandwagon. Try guava jelly on your toast instead of grape or apple jelly for an offbeat treat.

22 Snack on cornstarch before bedtime.

Uncooked cornstarch (UCS) is a complex carbohydrate that gets digested and absorbed slowly, providing a steady source of glucose for up to seven hours. Research shows eating UCS as part of a bedtime snack may protect you from morning bouts of low blood sugar (hypoglycemia). That was the case for diabetics in one study who drank UCS dissolved in a non-sugary drink, like milk or sugar-free soda, before bedtime. But you don't have to mix your own cornstarch drink. Manufacturers now make diabetic snack bars with UCS, sold as Nite Bite, Extend Bar, and Gluc-O-Bar. Experts say eating them before bedtime, during long bouts between meals, after exercise, and after drinking alcohol may help prevent hypoglycemia. Keep in mind that none of these snacks are meant to treat emergency hypoglycemia because they don't digest fast enough.

A Closer Look
Dodging diabetes

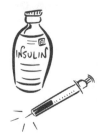

America keeps getting fatter, and that extra weight means more cases of diabetes. You develop diabetes when your body can't properly produce or use insulin. This hormone helps your cells transform food into energy for everyday life.

Diabetes already ranks as the sixth leading cause of death in the United States — and it's on the rise. From 1970 to 2002, deaths from diabetes jumped 45 percent, while those from heart disease and stroke declined. Fortunately, diet and lifestyle changes can help reduce your risk for diabetes — and help you control it if you already have it.

Dangers of diabetes

Diabetes comes in two main categories, but the second is much more common.

▸ Type 1, also known as juvenile or insulin dependent diabetes, is an autoimmune disease which usually strikes people under the age of 30. Your body does not produce insulin, so you need to inject it.

▸ Type 2, also called adult onset or non-insulin dependent diabetes, accounts for 90 to 95 percent of all cases. It often affects overweight, inactive people.

If you have type 2 diabetes, your body probably makes enough insulin but has "forgotten" how to use it. Your cells have become resistant to insulin so the glucose from the food you eat builds up in your blood instead of nourishing your cells.

High blood sugar levels can start an avalanche of other medical problems, including high cholesterol and high blood pressure. Type 2 diabetics risk blindness, amputations, kidney disease, heart disease, strokes, and nerve damage.

Symptoms of diabetes include frequent urination, excessive thirst or increased appetite, unexplained weight loss, and blurry vision. Seniors, blacks, Latinos, Native Americans, and Asians have an increased risk. You're also more at risk if it's in your family or you're overweight.

Smart eating strategies

Diet becomes extremely important when you have diabetes. You won't find a magic, one-size-fits-all diabetes diet, but you can discover the best plan for you by working with a registered dietitian or certified diabetes educator. Your goal is to keep your blood sugar from getting too high or too low. In general, you want to stick to a healthy diet with a good balance of carbohydrates, protein, and fats.

Make room for whole grains and starches, fruits, vegetables, low-fat or nonfat milk, lean meat, poultry, and fish, cheese, and beans. Specific foods, like cinnamon and coffee, may also help. Limit saturated fats, sweets, and alcohol. Eat high-fat or sugary foods like potato chips, crackers, cookies, candy, and fried foods only once in a while.

Portion control is key to managing your diabetes — and your weight. Be sure you understand serving sizes. Weigh and measure your food, if you need to. Eating roughly the same amount of food at the same time each day helps keep your blood sugar steady. Stick to a schedule for meals and snacks, and do not skip meals.

Helpful steps

Recent studies show that a 30-minute brisk walk each day can dramatically lower your blood pressure as well as help you lose weight, reduce stress, and even treat diabetes by reducing your need for insulin or drugs. Boost your daily walk to an hour, and you can cut your risk of type 2 diabetes in half. Here are some other steps to take to prevent or control diabetes.

- **Lose weight.** Just dropping 10 to 20 pounds makes a big difference. For best results, combine a low-fat diet with an exercise program.

- **Take care of your feet.** Diabetic neuropathy, or nerve damage from high blood pressure, leads to about 54,000 foot amputations a year. Wear comfortable shoes, keep your feet clean and dry, and inspect them regularly for redness or sores, especially after exercise. Report problems to your doctor.

- **Consider aspirin therapy.** An aspirin a day can lower your risk of heart attack. At higher doses, aspirin reversed insulin resistance in overweight mice.

- **Get plenty of sleep.** People who don't get enough sleep are more likely to become resistant to insulin — a direct path to diabetes. Strive for at least eight hours of snooze time.

- **Skip the nightcap.** A drink before bed can be dangerous for some diabetics, causing a drop in blood sugar the next morning.

- **Brush and floss.** Gum disease makes it harder to control blood sugar.

- **Monitor your blood pressure and cholesterol.** You don't want heart problems to sneak up on you. Try to keep your LDL cholesterol below 100 and your HDL cholesterol above 45. Blood pressure should be at or below 130/85.

- **Quit smoking.** One study found that people who smoked 20 or more cigarettes a day were 70 percent more likely to develop diabetes than former smokers or those who never smoked.

Talk to your doctor about monitoring your blood sugar. He'll let you know how often to check and what your target levels should be at different times, such as before meals or bedtime.

Do your best to avoid diabetes. But if you have the disease, a healthy diet, regular exercise, and medication if needed, can help you live with it successfully.

Lower carbs to lower risk?

Carbohydrates have more effect on blood sugar than any other nutrient. So does it help to limit your carbs? A recent Temple University study of 10 obese people with type 2 diabetes found that a strict low-carb diet helped them lose weight and improve blood sugar levels. However, the study was small and strictly controlled, and the long-term effects of such a diet — high in protein and fat and low in fiber — remain unknown.

In fact, a recent Harvard study shows that the iron from red meat can lead to type 2 diabetes. And there are concerns about a high-protein diet's effect on your kidneys — not to mention your heart and arteries. Your best bet is to talk to your doctor before beginning a low-carbohydrate, high-protein diet.

Cancer fighters

28 foods to keep cancer at bay

Just three simple changes could prevent up to 4 million cases of cancer every year worldwide, suggests a report from the American Institute of Cancer research. Those three changes? Eat right, exercise, and maintain an appropriate weight. The report adds that just a little more than 14 ounces of a variety of fruits and veggies daily could prevent 20 percent of cancer cases. That's just three to four half-cup servings.

But some foods, or the way you cook them, may actually put you more at risk for cancer. Moreover, studies suggest that vitamin and mineral deficiencies can raise cancer risk. So it pays to eat the right foods to prevent vitamin and mineral shortfalls and avoid cancer-causing substances.

And you'll get a bonus for doing it. The best foods also contain incredible natural compounds that defend your body against cancer. Antioxidants protect you from faulty free radical molecules that can help cancer ignite. These faulty molecules can be created as your body processes the oxygen you breathe, so you need plenty of antioxidants. Many phytonutrients or phytochemicals are also cancer fighters. You'll find these naturally occurring chemicals in spices, grains, nuts, beans, fruits, and vegetables.

1 **Fight off tumors with blueberry bodyguards.** Blueberries are full of antioxidants like anthocyanins and ellagic acid. Antioxidants are tough on cancer because oxidation spurs on the development of this disease. Think of it this way. If you slice an apple, it turns brown. But a little lemon juice applied to the cut surface prevents the apple from becoming discolored. When these antioxidants intervene inside your body, they also prevent oxidation from damaging cells — and reduce the risk of cancer. No wonder blueberries are causing so much excitement. Top yogurt, cereal, or ice cream with blueberries, or add them to salads, muffins, or pancakes.

2 **Discover the antioxidant mother lode in mushrooms.** Scientists thought wheat germ and chicken livers were top sources of the potent, cell-protecting antioxidant ergothioneine. But now they say plain old button mushrooms can give you at least four times as much ergothioneine as wheat or chicken. In fact, you could get up to 5 milligrams just by adding 3 ounces of white button mushrooms to your favorite salad or pizza — a mere handful or two. Switch to 3 ounces of maitake or shiitake mushrooms to get more than twice the white button ergothioneine — and hearty portabella mushrooms deliver the most of all. Stubborn and powerful, ergothioneine even stays in mushrooms after you cook them.

New!

Coming soon to a supermarket near you — yellow, pink, purple, and green rice — all colored by healthy phytonutrients. The yellow rice draws its color from curcumin, a golden plant chemical that may fight inflammation and cancer. Tomatoes tint the pink rice. The purple and green rices gain their hue from wholesome vegetables. You may pay a little extra for these rices, but you'll get extra nutrition, too.

3 **Block cancer with broccoli sprouts.** These baby bloomers are even more potent than the adult version. Three-day-old broccoli sprouts have 20 to 50 times more sulforaphane — a promising cancer fighter — than regular broccoli. Brand new laboratory research suggests broccoli sprouts help stop bladder cancer. And animal tests have shown sulforaphane can block mammary, colon, and stomach tumors. Food-borne illness from bacteria, like *Salmonella* and *E. coli*, has been a concern with sprouts, but a product called Broccosprouts uses patented technology and strict sanitation guidelines to ensure safe sprouts. Ask about Broccosprouts at your favorite supermarket or health food store.

4 **Nab cereal's new weapon against cancer.** Remarkable new research suggests you can cut your risk of colon, breast, and ovarian cancer if you get enough vitamin D. Many cereals are fortified with this important vitamin, so check the label and choose your cereal wisely. Also try for a low-sugar or no-sugar cereal that is high in fiber. The extra fiber could help lower your risk of breast and colon cancer even more.

Daily Vitamin D

Over 50 — 10 mcg (400 IU)

Over 70 — 15 mcg (600 IU)

5 **Aim pomegranate juice at prostate cancer.** Pomegranate extract helps prevent prostate cancer in animals, a new laboratory study suggests. It also inhibits prostate cancer cell growth and encourages those cells to die. Although human research has not been done as yet, the study's researchers say drinking pomegranate juice can't hurt and might help. For a unique way to enjoy pomegranate juice, soften up the pomegranate by rolling it on your counter. Then poke a hole in the top, stick a straw in, and drink up.

6 **Get extra defense from garlic.** Just season processed meats with this pungent spice. Nitrites used to preserve these meats may become cancer-causing nitrosamines, but garlic can help prevent that. As if that's not enough, garlic's allicin and sulfur compounds rev up your immune system to blast tumors and cancer cells. Allylsulfides even turn cancer-causing substances water soluble to help your body sweep them out. Research suggests that people who load up on garlic may have less risk of stomach and esophageal cancer than garlic-haters. Studies have also shown a link between eating garlic and a reduced risk of colon, prostate, bladder, skin, and lung cancer.

7 **"Soup" up pancreas and prostate protection.** And make it tomato soup. A Canadian study found that a diet rich in tomatoes and tomato products helps reduce the risk of deadly pancreatic cancer. This diet could cut prostate cancer risk, too. Scientists think lycopene, a phytonutrient in tomatoes, may be the key to tomato's anti-cancer powers. While they investigate, enjoy delicious treats like tomato soup, marinara with vegetables, salsa, or sun-dried tomatoes.

Top non-tomato lycopene sources

▸ watermelon

▸ pink or red grapefruit

▸ sweet red pepper

▸ cooked asparagus

▸ red cabbage

8 **Enjoy a bag of Brazil nuts.** You may help your body resist cancers of the esophagus, lung, stomach, colon and rectum. That's because Brazil nuts are a powerhouse of the anti-cancer nutrient selenium. In fact, the National Cancer Institute thinks something in Brazil nuts may safeguard you from cancer. That's why they're funding a 12-year study of 30,000 men to learn whether selenium, vitamin E, or both help prevent prostate cancer. Meanwhile, you can add a few Brazil nuts to a salad or snack — or get selenium from other sources like broccoli, cabbage, celery, chicken, eggs, garlic, milk, mushrooms, and bran.

Asian diet may hold anti-cancer secrets

Many types of cancer that plague the rest of the world are uncommon in Asia. Following these steps in the Asian diet pyramid may help you avoid cancer, too.

▸ Eat high-fiber grains like rice at nearly every meal.

▸ Eat fruits, nuts, beans, seeds, and plenty of fresh vegetables daily.

▸ Include small amounts of vegetable oil, fish, shell-fish, and dairy products every day.

▸ Eat sweets, eggs, and poultry only weekly, and red meat, just once a month.

▸ Cut the fat in cooking. Steam or stir-fry foods to keep the fat content low.

9 Get prevention in a walnut shell. A few walnuts a day may help prevent prostate cancer. A 59-country study found that nuts, along with grains and cereals, help shield you. Besides, walnuts are a top natural source of ellagic acid, a flavonoid that fights cancers of the lung, liver, skin, and esophagus. Just remember these two caveats about these tasty nuts. They're a common source of food allergies, and their load of healthy fats means you can gain weight if you eat too many.

10 Slice your risk of cancer with cantaloupe. New research suggests you can do it if you get more beta carotene and other carotenoids from foods like cantaloupe. Scientists have also found that people

Bonus cancer-blasting phytochemicals	
Antioxidant	**Foods to eat**
lutein	corn, spinach, tomatoes, broccoli, oranges, cabbage, kale
alpha carotene	carrots, pumpkin
beta cryptoxanthin	oranges, cooked pumpkin, sweet red peppers, papaya, tangerines
quercetin	onions, apples
naringin	white grapefruit
ferulic acid	cooked corn

whose diets are rich in cantaloupe's beta carotene have a lower risk of cancers of the head, neck, mouth, uterus, prostate, and blood. The National Cancer Institute and USDA recommend 5.2 to 6 milligrams of beta carotene daily, but most Americans get far less. A single cup of cantaloupe has 3.6 milligrams. You'll get more of it from deep, dark-fleshed melons than from paler ones.

11 Use old bean for new cancer defender.

Scientists already knew about the inositol pentakisphosphate in lima beans — but now animal and laboratory research suggests it may inhibit the growth of cancer cells and may even make anti-cancer drugs more effective. Although more research is needed, regularly serving up hot lima beans as a side dish couldn't hurt.

12 **Lower risk with cabbage.** A new study suggests eating cabbage — or one of its family members — at least once a week means extra lung cancer protection for most of us. But that's not all. Researchers say this inexpensive vegetable can also help prevent cancer of the colon, brain, breast, stomach, and bladder. It's also ultra low-calorie and has ultra high cancer-fighting nutrients like high voltage indoles, mighty glucosinolates, cancer-preventing sulforaphane and other isothiocyanates. And if you hate that "cooked cabbage" smell, boil it in anything but aluminum pots and pans, and try cabbage siblings like cauliflower or brussels sprouts.

13 **Gain double defense from sweet peppers.** First, the antioxidant powers of vitamin C in these peppers may save you from cancers of the stomach, throat, lung, bladder, and pancreas. Second, if you have an ulcer, you can eat these to avoid the acidity of citrus fruits that may bother your belly. Other gentle sources of vitamin C include strawberries, broccoli, cantaloupe, and brussels sprouts.

14 **Fight two cancers with broccoli.** Meet indole-3-carbinol, a natural cancer foe in broccoli. University of California scientists claim this powerful chemical stops the growth of breast cancer cells. And a new animal study adds that the isothiocyanates in broccoli may also help ax lung cancer risk in smokers and former smokers. Those are two good reasons to enjoy more of this healthy veggie. But try to avoid boiling or microwaving broccoli as the water leaches out cancer-fighting nutrients. Surprisingly, one study found that broccoli loses up to 97 percent of some antioxidants when microwaved. Instead steam broccoli, or choose a speedy cooking technique that uses little water.

15 **Seize more protection with turmeric.** This spice contains curcumin, a golden antioxidant that may help prevent eight types of cancers — lung, blood, breast, stomach, colon, mouth, skin, and liver. And new research shows that high doses of curcumin rev up the short-term death rate of melanoma skin cancer cells while low doses push up these cells' long-term death rates. To boost your protection, try a pepper-laced Thai curry dish with some green tea. The pepper and tea might help you absorb 20 times more curcumin. But if that's too spicy, just use turmeric to liven up mayonnaise, cream sauces, beans, or rice.

Don't forget anti-cancer spices

Many spices can boost your anti-cancer diet. Here's how they help.

▸ Ginger and chili — help keep tumors from forming

▸ Coriander — fights substances that help cause cancer

▸ Fennel, caraway, tarragon, and cumin — help block tumors from growing

▸ Saffron and paprika — rev up immunity

Anise, turmeric, rosemary, thyme, oregano, and sage may also help prevent cancer, according to the National Cancer Institute.

16 **Wield olive oil against breast cancer.** According to a new study, oleic acid, a monounsaturated fatty acid in olive oil, targets the main gene that promotes breast cancer. In fact, a Harvard research study reported that Greek women who consumed olive oil more than once a day had lower breast cancer odds than women who ate it less often. Try replacing meats, cheeses, and heavy sauces in your diet with olive oil-laced salad dressings, sauces, and Mediterranean dishes.

17 **Tap turnip greens to sidestep colon cancer.** New research of more than 45,000 women shows that those who consumed the most calcium had a lower risk of colon cancer than those who got the least. If you don't care for dairy foods, turnip greens are a good substitute. A cup of chopped turnip greens delivers 249 mg of calcium — more than 6 ounces of skim milk. Add chopped turnip greens to your next stir-fry dish for a calcium boost.

18 **Slash colon cancer risk with barley.** You may cut your risk by 40 percent if you raise your daily fiber intake from 15 grams to 35. Soluble fiber, the main kind in oat bran and barley, may react with the tiny organisms in your large intestine to form compounds that safeguard your colon. Both also speed stool through your body, which helps protect against constipation as well as cancer. Plus, the indigestible resistant starches in barley seem to fight off cancer-causing substances in the colon. For the most fiber and nutrients, bypass the pale or whitish heavily pearled barley, and look for lightly pearled barley. It's roughly the color of brown rice.

Watch out!

A new study suggests that diets high in refined sugars and starches may increase your risk of breast cancer. Research also shows that limiting salt and salty foods may help prevent gastric cancer. Trade empty calorie snacks and junk food for cancer-preventing foods you enjoy.

19 **Include black beans in your diet.** Eating them or other legumes at least three times a week may slice the risk of colon cancer for red meat lovers, scientists say. Black beans have natural cancer fighters called lignans and health-building phytochemicals like anthocyanins — the famous nutrients in blueberries and blackberries. Even better, these delicious beans are also high in the indigestible resistant starch that helps fend off colon cancer. So mix up black beans with rice and diced tomatoes, or enjoy hearty black bean soup.

20 **Eat three servings of sauerkraut a week.** You'll be less likely to get breast cancer than women who eat this food once a week or less, new research shows. During the pickling process that ferments white cabbage into sauerkraut, potent cancer-fighting isothiocyanates are created. These phytochemicals rev up anti-cancer enzymes and are particularly effective against lung and breast cancers. Eat sauerkraut plain, in salads, or along with other foods. Just remember to rinse and drain it before serving to ease up on the sodium.

21 **Pile on protection from black raspberries.** Scientists are testing a freeze-dried black raspberry powder that may deliver more cancer fighting nutrients than you can get from eating the berries. But that doesn't mean you shouldn't eat raspberries anymore. Their ellagic acid may help prevent four kinds of cancer — lung, liver, skin, and esophagus. In addition, a new laboratory study reports that two more compounds in black raspberry inhibit the growth of cancer cells — ferulic acid and beta sitosterol. So keep eating black raspberries and keep an eye out for that freeze-dried powder.

22

Cripple cancer causers with strawberries.
These berries are a good source of pectin — a surprising cancer foe. Research shows that rats fed a 10-percent pectin diet had a 50-percent plummet in colon cancer. Scientists think pectin may cripple cancer-causing agents in the colon. To get the results seen in the research, you'd need to eat piles of produce — up to 15 apples a day. Yet you can still get some defense if you eat strawberries and other pectin sources like apples, grapefruit, oranges, tangerines, and prunes. Add the fruits to desserts, or check your health food store for powdered fruit pectin. You can add a couple of teaspoons to baked goods.

TIP
Cooking

Replace a tenth of your ground meat with cherries before grilling, and you'll cut cancer-causing substances by up to 90 percent. Or marinade your meat first, using a flavoring like garlic or onion, a base (honey or oil), and an acidic liquid like lemon juice or vinegar.

23

Kill the big C with cranberries.
This berry's unusual proanthocyanidins trounced leukemia, colon cancer, and lung cancer cells in a recent laboratory study but left healthy cells untouched. Such compounds in cranberry may inhibit tumors and might even help prevent cancer cells from breaking loose to spread to new areas of the body, the study suggests. Although more research is needed, why not try cranberries — fresh or dried — in chicken salad, cereal, or rice? Or look for juice products with the highest percentage of cranberry juice and the least sugar or corn syrup.

24 **Find an ounce of peanut prevention.** That ounce of peanuts contains about as much cancer-threatening resveratrol as two pounds of grapes, claims the Peanut Institute. Resveratrol is a cancer-foiling antioxidant that fights inflammation, cell mutation, and tumors. A laboratory study even suggests resveratrol helps trigger the death of esophageal cancer cells. Peanuts are a common source of allergies, but you can substitute other resveratrol-rich foods — like grapes, grape juice, and, occasionally, wine — if you need to avoid allergic reactions.

25 **Bring in green tea reinforcements.** Thanks to powerful polyphenols called catechins, drinking green tea regularly could cut your risk of esophageal cancer by up to 50 percent. It could also lower your odds of stomach, gastrointestinal, liver, lung, and pancreatic cancers. And new research suggests two cups of black or green tea a day may cut ovarian cancer risk by up to 46 percent. Don't steep green tea for longer than two minutes or black tea for longer than five. Longer steeping adds bitter tannins and may limit your ability to absorb iron.

26 **Live longer with tantalizing apricots.** An Asian mountain tribe that eats apricots regularly has no history of health problems like cancer, heart disease, high blood pressure, and high cholesterol. This phenomenon has led some to believe this delectable fruit may be the secret to long life. Research has shown the beta carotene in apricots could cut your odds of some stomach and intestinal cancers. Plus their B vitamins may protect you from Alzheimer's and age-related memory loss. Peel and slice fresh apricots in yogurt or on ice cream, or eat dried ones as a sweet snack.

27 **Neutralize toxic substances with asparagus.** The antioxidant glutathione may help defend against disease and cell damage, and that makes it an effective cancer fighter. Although your body makes glutathione, you can also get it from fresh fruits and vegetables like asparagus. Of 15 vegetables tested for glutathione, researchers in Turkey found asparagus had the most by far. Processed foods, like canned vegetables, contain less glutathione than fresh ones, so choose fresh asparagus to get the richest source of this powerful antioxidant.

28 **Add beets, subtract risk.** Slice just a half cup of sunshine-fresh beets into a big salad and you'll get almost a fifth of the daily folate doctors recommend. That's good news because folate deficiency can raise your risk for a perilous pile of cancers — including cancer of the brain, lung, cervix, esophagus, pancreas, breast, and rectum. What's more, new research suggests that getting more folate cuts your colon cancer odds — especially if you smoke. For extra folate, eat dark leafy greens, legumes, seeds, and enriched breads and cereals.

A Closer Look
Combating carcinogens

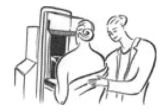

When it comes to cancer, there is good news and bad news.

First, the bad news. Cancer ranks as the No. 2 cause of death in the United States, behind only heart disease. Now for the good news. Many cancers can be prevented with a healthy diet and lifestyle.

Find out what causes cancer and what steps you can take to reduce your risk.

Cells gone wild

Cancer is a disease marked by abnormal, out-of-control cell growth. It begins with a single cell that has divided abnormally and does not function as it should. Because altered body cells multiply at an abnormally fast rate, they disrupt and destroy the normal function of the tissue or organs where they grow. If not held in check, cancer can spread throughout your body, destroying other organs and body tissues.

For women, breast cancer is the most common cancer, while prostate cancer is most likely to strike men. However, lung cancer kills more people than any other cancer. While some cancers run in the family, most come from outside factors. Cancer-causing substances, called carcinogens, trigger the process. Carcinogens include certain chemicals and viruses, but many crop up in foods and other lifestyle choices.

Beware of carcinogens

You can't avoid every carcinogen in the world. In fact, small amounts of carcinogens appear in everyday foods like coffee and toast. Don't worry — your body can handle these tiny amounts. But you can limit your exposure to other carcinogens if you alter your cooking methods, make smart food choices, and change some bad habits.

Grill with caution. Everyone loves a good barbecue. But watch out for charred foods. High-temperature cooking like grilling, broiling, and pan-frying causes heterocyclic amines (HCAs) to form. These potential carcinogens can lead to breast, stomach, and colorectal cancers. You may be able to lessen your risk by marinating your meat first. Also, line your grill with aluminum foil, and take care not to burn your food. An occasional steak or burger won't kill you, but try to limit grilled, fried, or smoked foods to once or twice a month.

Mind your meat. You'll also want to limit processed foods, like smoked, pickled, or cured meats. These salty foods may increase your risk of stomach cancer. Nitrites, found in bacon, hot dogs, and processed meats, form nitrosamines, a type of carcinogen.

Stop smoking. This nasty habit not only leads to lung cancer, but also boosts your risk for oral, throat, esophageal, stomach, liver, prostate, and colorectal cancers. Also, ditch the chewing tobacco, and try to stay away from secondhand smoke.

Shield the sun. Too much exposure to the sun or tanning booths can increase your risk for skin cancer. Wear protective clothing, sunscreen, and sunglasses, and try to avoid the sun during the peak hours of 10 a.m. to 3 p.m.

Looking for more ways to reduce your cancer risk? Try these four simple steps from the American Cancer Society.

- Choose most of the foods you eat from plant sources. Load up on fruits and vegetables as well as breads, cereals, rice, pasta, and beans.

- Limit your intake of high-fat foods, especially from animal sources. Cut down on meat, especially fatty meat.

- Be physically active. Achieve and maintain a healthy weight. Aim for at least 30 minutes of moderate exercise a day.

- Limit consumption of alcoholic beverages, if you drink at all. That means one drink a day for a woman and two for a man.

A smart diet, sensible exercise program, and healthy habits can help keep you cancer-free. But, unless you take added precautions, cancer can still sneak up on you.

Tests are best

How can you tell if you have cancer? Often, you can't. Don't wait until it's too late. Early detection often means the difference between life and death. Go to your doctor for regular screenings.

Here is a look at the tests you might undergo for various cancers and how often you should be tested. If you have a personal or family history of cancer, you might opt for earlier and more frequent tests.

- **Breast cancer.** In addition to monthly self exams for lumps or other warning signs, you should have a mammogram every year after age 40.

- **Colon cancer.** When you turn 50, get serious about colon cancer screening. Options include a fecal occult blood test or fecal immunochemical test every year, a flexible sigmoidoscopy or double-contrast barium enema every five years, and a colonoscopy every 10 years.

- ▸ **Cervical cancer.** Get an annual Pap smear beginning no later than age 21. After age 30 — and three normal tests in a row — you can get screened every two to three years. When you reach age 70, you can opt to stop screening as long as you have had three normal tests in a row and no abnormal results in the past 10 years.

- ▸ **Prostate cancer.** Men age 50 and older should get an annual prostate-specific antigen (PSA) blood test and digital rectal examination. Those at high risk should begin testing at age 45 or even 40.

Also, make sure to report any symptoms of cancer to your doctor right away. These include lumps in the breast, changes to a wart or mole, sores that don't heal, a nagging cough or hoarseness, changes in bowel or bladder habits, indigestion or difficulty swallowing, unexplained changes in weight, and unusual bleeding or discharge.

Menu for avoiding cancer

Just as important as avoiding or limiting certain foods is eating the right ones. Make room on your plate for these foods with cancer-fighting properties.

- ▸ Fruits and vegetables, especially cruciferous vegetables and citrus fruits, for their antioxidants and phytonutrients

- ▸ Yogurt, for probiotics

- ▸ Tea, which has catechins

- ▸ Flaxseed, rich in lignans and fiber

- ▸ Tomatoes and tomato products, for lycopene

- ▸ Onions and garlic, which contain sulfur compounds

- ▸ Whole grains, for fiber and selenium

A+ 'regulators'

17 foods that set your system straight

Being regular means having timely and trouble-free bowel movements. It's not a pleasant topic of conversation, but not being regular is even more unpleasant. Fortunately, you can make food choices that help you stay regular and eliminate the need to talk about it.

Diarrhea is at one end of the irregularity scale. You're likely to have it about four times a year. It usually lasts a couple of days and goes away by itself. If it happens more than that, you need to see a doctor.

Constipation is at the other end. It's uncomfortable and can cause hemorrhoids and diverticulitis. Irritable bowel syndrome (IBS) may involve both constipation and diarrhea. Sometimes called spastic colon, IBS adds bloating and abdominal pain to its list of unpredictable bowel habits.

Many people don't realize how important diet is in keeping regular. Few get the American Dietetic Association's recommended 20 to 35 grams of fiber a day. They eat too many processed foods and not enough natural fruits, vegetables, and grains. Fiber adds bulk and softens your stool and also keeps it moving through your system.

Stress, bacteria, reactions to food or medicines, and lactose intolerance also may cause irregularity. And other nutrients besides fiber can help straighten you out. Here are a few foods that will keep your digestive tract on track.

1 **Fight diarrhea with bananas.** The dehydration that comes with diarrhea robs you not only of fluids but vital minerals, too. Bananas are the perfect food after a diarrhea attack because they put those minerals back into your body. Bananas are the first part of the BRAT (Bananas, Rice, Applesauce, Toast) diet recommended as a transition back to regular food. They're rich in fiber but gentle and bland enough to pass through your weakened digestive tract. When you go places where sanitary conditions may foster traveler's diarrhea, avoid dangerous bacteria by eating bananas and other foods you can peel.

2 **Keep fluids with chocolate.** New research verifies an ancient European and South American practice of treating diarrhea with cocoa. A recent study discovered that certain flavonoids in cocoa could limit the development of fluids that cause diarrhea. Scientists hope to use these flavonoids to create natural supplements that will cut down on diarrhea symptoms. In the meantime, see if some dark chocolate doesn't help the next time you have an attack. It has to be dark chocolate, though, which has high concentrations of cocoa. Some chocolate has a lot less cocoa and therefore not as many of those helpful flavonoids.

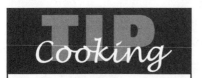

Cooking TIP

Canned vegetables sometimes have more fiber than fresh ones, but the added salt is a problem. Pour off the water and rinse foods like beans and vegetables before you cook them to get rid of the excess sodium.

3 **Cure everything with rhubarb.** Low doses of rhubarb root extract seem to relieve diarrhea, while higher amounts help keep you regular. That's because rhubarb contains phytochemicals called phenols and tannins. Phenols have a laxative effect, and tannins help curb diarrhea. The edible rhubarb stalks have the same phytochemicals, plus they're loaded with fiber, vitamins, and minerals. Rhubarb also stimulates gastric juices and improves your digestion.

4 **Pick pineapple for double duty.** Some nutritionists think eating just 4 ounces of pineapple a day may be enough to cure constipation. This juicy tropical fruit is also a source of bromelain, an enzyme that seems to treat and prevent diarrhea caused by *Escherichia coli* bacteria. Food poisoning from *E. coli* is one of the more common and dangerous ways to come down with diarrhea. Experts suggest higher doses of bromelain supplement for the best prevention, but a little extra protection from a bowl of fresh pineapple isn't a bad idea. Pineapple juice or canned pineapple won't help, however. They don't contain active bromelain.

> **TIP**
> *Buying*
>
> A quick way to get fresh, nutritious vegetables on your table is to buy pre-packaged salad ingredients. Look for a mixture of vegetables already cut, washed, chopped and ready to serve. Your store may also have a fresh salad or deli bar, where you can choose your own combinations and quantities.

5 **Stay regular with apples.** Whether your problem is visiting the bathroom too much or not enough, an afternoon apple snack may be your simple solution. This juicy fruit can fix both diarrhea and constipation. A single unpeeled apple contains up to 5 grams of fiber, the most

Types of fiber		
	Insoluble	**Soluble**
Characteristics	Does not dissolve	Dissolves in water
Action	Adds bulk; speeds up trip through your digestive system	Makes food soft and gummy so it moves through your system easier
Best sources	Oats, rye, barley, peas, beans, citrus fruits, pectin, psyllium	Whole-wheat breads & cereals, brown rice, beans, popcorn, celery, corn

important nutrient for keeping your bowels working right. Apples contain pectin, a soluble fiber that absorbs water in your stomach and intestines. It moistens, softens, and swells your stool to help out difficult bowel movements. Pectin also firms up the watery stool of diarrhea, changing it to a thicker consistency. Applesauce is another part of the BRAT diet for diarrhea recovery. Just watch out for the extra sweeteners in some brands of applesauce. They can make your diarrhea worse instead of better.

6 **Depend on cereal, not laxatives.** You can become dependent on laxatives if you use them too often. They can lose their effectiveness and actually cause constipation. Other side effects of laxative overuse are cramping, diarrhea, and dehydration. Instead of making your problems worse, turn to natural solutions like whole-grain cereals with fiber to soften and bulk up your stools and keep them moving properly. Just take time to read the fine print when choosing a cereal. Names can be misleading, so look for the fiber content. You can find bran flakes that range from 4 to 12 grams of fiber per serving. Some cereals are also loaded with sugar but have

little or no fiber. Raisin bran is one of your best bets because you get fiber from both the bran and the raisins.

7 **Don't forget about prunes.** They call them dried plums so you'll think about all the other things they are good for besides curing constipation. But dried plums are still one of the best natural laxatives you can find. They have lots of fiber, plus other natural laxative power from things like phenolic compounds and sorbitol. A California study found that men who ate 12 dried plums a day increased their stool volume by 20 percent and did not get diarrhea. Most of the fiber in dried plums is pectin, which helps firm things up to relieve diarrhea. Eat dried plums right out of the box, or mix them into cookies or pancakes. Cut down on fat by substituting prune puree for oil in baked goods.

8 **Turn to beans to ditch diverticulosis.** You get diverticulosis when the pressure and straining of chronic constipation pushes out little sacs or pouches in your intestinal

Avoid these troublemakers

If you have diverticulosis, these things can make it worse.

- High-protein diets — you lose out on fiber-rich fruits, vegetables, and whole grains.

- Refined grains — processing strips out the fiber.

- Red meat — bacteria formed when you digest red meat weakens intestinal walls. The fat also increases your risk.

- Stimulant laxatives — they irritate your colon more than they help. Use natural laxatives instead.

- Seeded foods — kernels and seeds may get caught in the little pockets.

wall. When bits of food and bacteria get trapped in these bubbles, you can end up with the infection, fever, and severe pain of diverticulitis. About a third of every North American over age 45 already has diverticulosis, but doctors and nutritionists think you can avoid it by eating foods high in fiber. Fiber keeps things moving easily through your system and also helps clean out those pouches before they get infected. Just one cup of black beans gives you 29 grams of this super nutrient.

Dried blueberries help diarrhea

Dried blueberries have been used in Sweden for centuries as a diarrhea cure. Experts aren't sure if the phytochemicals in blueberries neutralize bacteria that cause diarrhea or if it's just the fiber that helps. If you can't find dried blueberries at your local market, you can make your own. Just spread some fresh berries out in the sun until they wrinkle and shrivel up. Eat about three tablespoons for a diarrhea attack, or crush them and make a tea.

9 **Collar constipation with cauliflower.** Not only is constipation uncomfortable, the pressure and straining it brings can cause hemorrhoids as well as diverticulosis. The best way to prevent and treat hemorrhoids is to prevent constipation. And the best way to get things moving again is to add more fiber to your diet with vegetables like cauliflower. Raw or cooked, cauliflower is a great source of fiber — a natural laxative that softens your stool to prevent constipation, which in turn takes the pressure off your hemorrhoids.

10 **Start your day with blueberries.** It's a delicious way to add fiber — a sure-fire remedy for constipation, which can lead to diverticular disease and hemorrhoids. Blueberries are great on breakfast cereal, with yogurt, or in a fruit cup. Fix blueberry muffins or pancakes for a special treat. A single cup of blueberries has 3.5 grams of fiber — about 15 percent of your recommended daily intake.

11 **Add water to your fiber.** If you're still constipated despite eating a lot of fiber-rich foods, you may need more water. Water helps fiber soften your stools and move them through your digestive tract. Without water, the extra fiber you eat could jam up and form an intestinal blockage, which is far worse than simple constipation. Water is especially important if you have diverticulosis because it helps flush out food and other particles that stick in your intestines. The old rule of six to eight glasses of water a day still makes a lot of sense.

12 **Eat an artichoke to ease IBS.** Artichoke leaf extract has been found to soothe irritable bowel syndrome (IBS). Final results are still pending, but eating artichokes could bring you some relief from the difficult digestive symptoms that make up IBS. Artichokes have a good amount of fiber *(see table)*, vitamin C, and phytochemicals that stimulate bile production to help digest fat and cholesterol. Cook artichokes by steaming or boiling for about 30 minutes. Eat the meaty part at the base of each leaf by

Serving	Fiber	Women's DRI	Men's DRI
1 medium artichoke	6.5 g	31%	22%
1/2 cup hearts	4.5 g	21%	15%

pulling it gently through your teeth. After the leaves are gone, you're left with the heart of the artichoke — a soft, nutty center that can be eaten whole after you scrape off the soft fuzz covering it.

13 **Enjoy papaya, a tropical treat.** Unripe papayas are abundant in papain, a unique enzyme that breaks down protein and is used in meat tenderizers. As this juicy fruit ripens, the papain weakens and becomes a mild digestive aid. Papayas are also rich in fiber and a host of antioxidants, so they should help soothe your uncomfortable IBS symptoms. Slice a ripe papaya and eat it like a melon, or cut it up and use it in fruit salad. Too much papain can be a problem, so cook unripe papayas to cut the strength of this enzyme.

TIP Serving

For a nutritious, digestive-friendly breakfast, mix muesli into your yogurt. You'll get the calcium and good bacteria from yogurt along with nutrients and fiber from the muesli. Look for it at the grocery store, or make your own using rolled oats, fruit, and nuts.

14 **Use yogurt for bacterial balance.** Billions of helpful bacteria live in your intestines. They help digest your food and protect you from harmful germs. Sometimes a round of antibiotics or poor eating habits kill off these good bugs, and harmful bacteria take their place. The results are digestive problems ranging from simple diarrhea to the multiple symptoms of IBS and even more complex problems. Fortunately, yogurt is full of probiotics — good bacteria that ferment dairy products and then become powerful disease fighters inside your body. The more yogurt you eat, the more these good bugs crowd out the bad ones. Just make sure the label says "active cultures" so you know your yogurt has living bacteria. If not, it won't do much good.

15 **Check out chicory for prebiotics.** Non-digestible carbohydrates called fructo-oligosaccharides encourage and provide food for probiotics, the good bacteria in your gut. These nutrients — known as prebi-otics — help keep your probiotic levels up so you won't experience intestinal distress. Other elements of chicory help improve your appetite in addition to curbing constipation, diarrhea, and indigestion. Although chicory leaves can be eaten as greens, it's the roots that give this plant its most fame. Roasted chicory root added to coffee gives it a distinctive bitter, mellow taste. New Orleans and other parts of the South are particularly noted for their chicory-flavored coffee.

Tiny seeds soothe IBS

Psyllium seeds are a super source of soluble fiber, which can help ease irritable bowel syndrome symptoms. People with IBS tend to move food slowly through their intestines, but psyllium seeds absorb water, which helps your stools pass easier through your system. They also stimulate peristalsis, the muscular squeezing that pushes stools smoothly through your body. If you need some gentle help with regularity, try a bulking agent that contains psyllium.

16 **Cut asparagus early and often.** Asparagus is the first thing you can harvest from your garden in the spring, and under ideal conditions it grows so fast you need to pick new spears every day. If you don't grow this delicacy, you can buy it fresh, frozen, or canned. Any way you like it, it's another of those vegetables that gives you plenty of fiber — even after it's been cooked — to keep away constipation, hemorrhoids, and diverticulitis. As an added bonus, asparagus also contains prebiotic compounds that encourage the growth of helpful digestive bacteria.

17 **Drink almond milk.** Regular dairy milk may be the cause of your IBS, either because the extra fat triggers the symptoms or because you are truly lactose intolerant. If so, look for almond milk in your grocer's dairy case. It's not a new idea — almond milk has been around since the Middle Ages, when animal milk was virtually useless because of the lack of refrigeration. You can make your own almond milk by steeping a cup of ground almonds in two cups of boiling water and blending to the right consistency.

A Closer Look
Focus on fiber

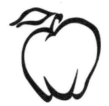

It's a bird, it's a plane, it's … fiber! This nutritional superhero can come to your rescue and keep you feeling good. Help yourself stay healthy by discovering the different types and sources of fiber and how to fit more of them into your diet.

Fiber facts

Fiber, also known as roughage, refers to the parts of fruits, vegetables, and grains that your body can't digest. There are two main kinds of fiber.

▸ **Soluble fiber.** This type of fiber turns soft and sticky in your body, slowing things down in your stomach and small intestine. This gives your body more time to whisk away bad cholesterol and absorb carbohydrates. Dried beans, peas, oats, barley, flaxseed, and many other fruits and vegetables contain soluble fiber.

▸ **Insoluble fiber.** The bulk of this fiber passes through your digestive system. It keeps your bowels moving smoothly and tones your digestive muscles. It also adds bulk to your stool and speeds it through the large intestine. This guards against constipation, diverticulosis, and possibly colon cancer. Look for insoluble fiber in whole-wheat foods, bran, and fruits and veggies with tough, chewy textures.

Ideally, you want to get a balance of soluble and insoluble fiber into your diet. You'll also probably want to up your fiber intake, because most people fall short of recommended levels. According to the Institute of Medicine, men over 50 should eat at least 30 grams of fiber each day, while women the same age should aim for 21 grams.

Fight disease with fiber

Why all the fuss about fiber? What makes it so great? Well, for starters, fiber can help you lose weight. The good news is that you can eat as much fiber as your body can handle. It has absolutely no calories, and what's more, your body needs it to function at its peak. Not only does fiber move through your system without adding calories, it also makes you feel full longer, so you're not snacking between meals. It may even block the absorption of some of the fat and protein you eat.

And because many high-fiber foods — like fruits and vegetables — are low in calories, you can actually eat more, not less, of many kinds of food and still lose weight and get healthy. Along with helping you stay in shape, fiber can help prevent conditions like constipation, hemorrhoids, diverticulosis, diabetes, heart attack, stroke, and cancer.

While fiber supplements are available, your best bet is to get your fiber from foods, which also contain lots of nutrients. Just make sure to add fiber to your diet gradually. Adding too much fiber too quickly can cause gas, abdominal cramps, bloating, and diarrhea. It's easy to find room for more fiber in your diet. Just replace some of your favorite low-fiber foods with high-fiber substitutes like these.

Instead of:	Eat:
orange juice	whole orange
cornflakes	raisin bran
white bread	bran muffin
white rice	brown rice
meat	beans
potato chips, other snacks	carrots, celery sticks
regular cookies	whole-grain cookies

Nausea relief

14 foods to ease the queasies

Most people have felt nauseous at some point in their lives. It's no fun. Nausea is an uneasy feeling in your stomach, which sometimes leads to vomiting. Along with an upset stomach, symptoms may include fever, sweat, chills, weakness, unnatural paleness, cramps, dry heaves, and an unusual amount of saliva.

If you eat food contaminated with viruses, parasites, pesticides, or bacteria like *E. coli*, you could experience severe nausea along with diarrhea, fever, and chills. Symptoms can show up within hours of eating contaminated food or even several days later. The germs that cause food poisoning are everywhere, but they're most abundant in meat, poultry, eggs, and milk.

If you're prone to motion sickness, one bumpy ride in a car, boat, or plane could lead to that dizzy, unconnected feeling.

Many other things can make you feel sick to your stomach, including infection, illness, vertigo, and food intolerances. But some things — particularly foods — can actually make you feel better. Here are some top choices for settling your stomach.

1 **Make bananas your first choice.** When your stomach is upset, pamper it with foods that won't make things worse. It's not complicated. Just follow the BRAT diet — foods that are bland and soft enough on your stomach that you'll be able to keep them down. The B in BRAT stands for bananas, the first food you should think of when you are not feeling well.

2 **Cook up some rice.** The R in BRAT stands for rice. It's a filling and nutritious dish that will stay in your stomach without causing trouble. Don't add spices or butter to it, though. The grease and spices would be too hard on your tummy.

TIP
Cooking

Keep a box of Rice Expressions frozen organic rice in your cupboard for days when your stomach is under the weather. Just pull out a pouch of rice and pop it in the microwave for 3 minutes. You'll have a hearty, stomach-friendly snack in no time. Look for Rice Expressions at natural food stores.

3 **Dig into applesauce.** The A in BRAT is a nice treat when you can only eat bland foods. Welcome the sweet taste of applesauce as a break from your meals of rice and bananas.

4 **Munch on toast.** Throw some bread in the toaster when your stomach can handle something more filling. Plain toast without butter makes a good snack, and toast completes the list of safe foods that make up the BRAT diet. When you do start feeling better, add more soft, bland foods like cooked cereal, eggs, custard, yogurt, soda crackers, skinless baked potatoes, or skinless chicken.

5 **Sip on soft drinks.** Take tiny sips of your favorite soft drink to settle an upset stomach. Small bits of clear, sweet liquids like soda and fruit juice can prevent vomiting. But don't drink orange juice or grapefruit juice

Nausea relief

because they're too acidic. For a double dose of nausea cure, drink ginger ale, preferably the natural kind made with real ginger. It will help relax the nerves and muscles in your digestive tract and put nausea to rest.

6 **Treat your stomach gingerly with ginger.** This spice has proven itself in study after study. It has cut off queasiness brought on by everything from motion sickness to chemotherapy and surgery. For your next trip, buy candied ginger at the supermarket or health food store. Eat two pieces — each roughly 1 inch by one-quarter inch thick — an hour before your departure. Then take the same amount every four hours during the voyage. Or try ginger capsules. You'll get the same dose from two 500-milligram pills. Ginger is also recommended for nausea caused by indigestion. Chop up a 1-inch piece of fresh ginger and boil it in hot water for 10 minutes to make a stomach-soothing tea.

7 **Send bacteria packing with dried plums.** Formerly known as prunes, dried plums still have the same fiber, vitamins, minerals,

Keep your produce squeaky clean

It's hard to believe, but you may have to worry more about catching a bacterial infection from produce than from meat. Fruits and vegetables make great homes for some of the worst guests, like *E. coli*, *Salmonella*, and *Listeria*. Wash your fruits and vegetables with water and rinse them thoroughly. Water can't guarantee 100 percent victory over bacteria, but it's your best bet. It's also a good idea to wash produce you plan to slice since your knife can spread bacteria from the skin to the insides of fruits and vegetables.

199

and antioxidants they had when they went by that other name. Their new image hasn't changed their antibacterial powers either. Studies show that dried plum puree will kill certain strains of bacteria that cause food poisoning. Just one tablespoon per pound of ground beef will kill up to 90 percent of *E. coli*, one of the most dangerous bacteria. It's nice to know you've got dried plums on your side.

> ## TIP
> ### Serving
>
> Make your usual cup of yogurt even healthier by adding your favorite fruit and a teaspoon of honey. For more fiber, grate the fruit with the peel before mixing it in. Fresh peaches, pears, and apples all work well. For an easy smoothie, put 8 ounces of plain non-fat yogurt in a glass or jar with 2 ounces of cold juice — fruit, tomato, or carrot juice will do — cover, and shake until smooth.

8 **Get friendly bacteria from yogurt.** Some bacteria work for you while others work against you. The good ones are called probiotics, and they help keep harmful bacteria in check. Yogurt has good bacteria, too, and if you eat this creamy dessert regularly, you'll add helpful bacteria to your digestive tract and possibly avoid intestinal problems. Research has shown for decades that yogurt can help treat and maybe even prevent intestinal infections caused by bacteria like *Salmonella* and *E. coli*.

9 **Sprinkle on the turmeric.** If something you've eaten is making you nauseous, turmeric might take care of that. This spice promotes production of bile in your digestive system, which helps you digest fat and hurry along the digestion process. The German Commission E, a world-famous authority on herbal medicine, suggests you take up to half a teaspoon daily to soothe an upset stomach. Sprinkle it into your own stir fries, or have a curry dish when you dine out. Turmeric is a big part of curry sauces.

10 **Fight food poisoning with garlic.** It contains allicin, a potent antibiotic that kills a variety of bacteria, viruses, fungi, molds, yeasts, and parasites. Some of garlic's victims include *H. pylori, Salmonella, Staphylococcus, E. coli,* and *Candida.* Allicin is so powerful that it appears to conquer some infections that normally stand up to antibiotics. This is helpful to remember when cooking hamburgers or other ground beef dishes. Researchers at Kansas State University discovered that adding 3 to 5 teaspoons of garlic powder to 2 pounds of ground beef may help protect you against *E. coli* poisoning.

TIP Kitchen

Save the time and energy it takes to peel garlic by hand. Stick garlic cloves in the microwave on high for 10 seconds, and watch the skins pop right off.

11 **Mix dry mustard into ground beef.** A recent study from Canada revealed that powdered mustard — also known as mustard flour or dry mustard — can kill *E. coli.* Scientists treated ground beef with mustard flour and then refrigerated it for several days. Depending on how much mustard flour was added, the *E. coli* was almost completely gone in as little as three days. A taste test revealed only a small difference in taste between meat treated with mustard flour and meat without. As long as you cook your meat thoroughly, there is only one rule — the more mustard flour you add beforehand, the quicker it kills *E. coli*. Look for dry mustard in the spice section of your local grocery store.

12 **Add onions to your burgers.** A Japanese study found that adding onions to ground beef helped neutralize *Salmonella,* a dangerous bacterium. As a bonus, onions even prevented the formation of potential cancer-causing compounds called heterocyclic amines. For tastier — and safer — burgers, just add a half-cup to one cup of chopped onion to each pound of ground beef you plan to grill.

Head off food poisoning

If you're having second thoughts about something you've eaten in a foreign country — like a salad or ice-filled drink — don't wait for food poisoning to kick in. Try to stop it before it starts. Pour yourself a glass of mineral water, and stir in 2 teaspoons of apple cider vinegar. If you're lucky, the vinegar will kill the bacteria before it's too late.

13 **Brew a cup of chamomile.** This plant has what scientists call antispasmodics — compounds that reduce spasms in your gastrointestinal tract. Chamomile is especially good for soothing anxiety, so it may also ease the tension that causes digestive problems like stomach cramps, gas, bloating, nausea, and indigestion. You can buy chamomile tea in any grocery store, or try making your own. Steep a heaping tablespoon of chamomile leaves in hot water in a covered container for 10 to 15 minutes. Then strain and drink. Just be careful if you have pollen allergies. You may also be allergic to chamomile.

14 Spice up your food with horseradish.

Horseradish and wasabi, otherwise known as Japanese horseradish, are two popular spices. They both may kill harmful bacteria in foods because they have an ingredient called allylisothiocyanate (AIT) that shows up when the spices are grated. AIT prevents growth of bacteria and fungi that cause food poisoning. Lab tests show that AIT works just as well at killing those microbes when it comes from horseradish and wasabi. If you can stand their potent flavor, you'll benefit from their protection.

Watch out!

Don't get carried away when you visit rural areas. If someone offers you fresh cow milk, just say no. Unpasteurized milk has lots of bacteria known to cause food illnesses. *Campylobacter*, the leading cause of diarrheal disease in the United States, also turns up in raw milk. Play it safe, and stick with pasteurized.

A Closer Look
Recipe for food safety

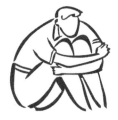

It's a jungle out there. Bacteria, parasites, viruses, and toxic chemicals can turn your kitchen — and your dinner — into a danger zone. Foodborne illness, or food poisoning, occurs when you eat contaminated food. It can leave you feeling awful. In some cases, it can even kill you.

Sources and symptoms

Bacteria, which thrive between 40 degrees and 140 degrees Fahrenheit, are the most common cause of foodborne illness. Raw meat, poultry, fish, eggs, and unpasteurized milk often harbor bacteria, which may also show up on fresh produce. Parasites, and viruses like hepatitis A, can also cause problems, as can household cleaning products.

Symptoms of foodborne illness include diarrhea, abdominal cramps, fever, headache, vomiting, severe exhaustion, and sometimes blood or pus in the stools. Sometimes, you'll feel sick right away, but usually it takes a few days or even weeks for symptoms to develop. Luckily, illness rarely lasts more than a day or two.

However, food poisoning can be a life-and-death issue for young children, older adults, and those with certain conditions, including liver disease, diabetes, cancer, and immune disorders. If you have severe symptoms, see a doctor or get emergency help. For milder symptoms, make sure to drink plenty of liquids to replace the fluids lost through vomiting and diarrhea.

Shopping strategies

Food poisoning prevention begins at the grocery store. Follow these tips to avoid bringing trouble home with your groceries.

▸ Don't buy cans of food that are swollen or leaking, and watch out for jars that have cracks or loose or bulging lids.

▸ Check expiration dates on perishable items, especially meats and dairy products. For items you won't use up right away, select those with the latest "sell by" date.

▸ Be sure frozen foods are rock-solid and the packages aren't torn or crushed.

▸ Buy only refrigerated eggs. Peek inside the carton to be sure they are clean and have no cracks.

▸ Save items that spoil quickly — like meats and frozen foods — for last. If it will take an hour or more to get home, take along an ice chest to keep those foods cold.

Storage solutions

Once you get your food home, how you store it can make a big difference. Make sure to take these precautions.

▸ Keep your refrigerator cooled to 40 degrees Fahrenheit or less and your freezer at 0 degrees Fahrenheit or less. Immediately refrigerate or freeze perishable items.

▸ Make sure meats are wrapped so their juices don't leak onto other foods.

▸ Refrigerate foodstuffs like mayonnaise and ketchup after they are opened. Read the labels on any items you're unsure about. Throw out anything you've left at room temperature by mistake.

▸ Store potatoes in a cool, dry place but not in the refrigerator or under the sink. Throw out any that have turned green.

▸ Never store food items near cleaning products or other chemicals.

If you have a power outage, keep your refrigerator and freezer doors closed to keep the heat out and the cold in. Your refrigerator should stay cool for at least four to six hours, while a full freezer can stay cold for two days.

Cooking and cleaning clues

Handle and prepare food with care to avoid foodborne illness. Here are some simple steps to keep in mind.

▸ Thaw frozen foods in the refrigerator or microwave, not on the countertop. Marinate food in the refrigerator, too.

▸ Wash your hands with warm, soapy water for at least 20 seconds before and after handling raw meat. Clean cutting boards, knives, and other utensils in warm soapy water between uses.

▸ Clean up spilled juices with paper towels rather than a dishcloth or sponge that's likely to spread germs. Scrub countertops where meat has been prepared with a mixture of a tablespoon of chlorine bleach to one quart of water.

▸ Cook meats thoroughly, and serve them on a clean platter, never on the unwashed dish that held the raw meat.

▸ Rinse fresh fruits and vegetables under running water. Use a scrub brush to remove dirt, if necessary.

▸ Refrigerate leftovers right away. Throw out anything that has been sitting out for more than two hours.

When cooking in a microwave, make sure you use microwave-safe containers. Cover the dish with a lid or plastic wrap, but let some steam escape. Stir or rotate food midway through to eliminate cold spots where harmful bacteria can survive. If you defrost food in the microwave, cook it right away because some parts may have started cooking already. Follow these tips, and you'll help keep yourself and those around you safe from harm.

Tummy tamers

16 foods to quiet the rumbles

Heartburn, gas, bloating, indigestion, upset stomach — all too often, these problems trace back to the foods you eat. You don't have to live in discomfort. Just as certain foods trigger gas or heartburn, so others can calm a troublesome tummy, or prevent those rumbles in the first place.

High-acid foods like tomatoes trigger heartburn for many people, but a cup of ginger tea can put out that fire. Similarly, certain foods, like cabbage, are bound to give you gas, but something as simple as flavoring it with caraway seeds can beat that bloating. You may even suffer from hidden health problems like lactose intolerance without realizing it. There's nutritional help for that, too.

Why not get to the root of your tummy troubles — what you are or aren't eating. If your doctor has ruled out disease, try healing naturally with nutrition.

1 **End indigestion with artichokes.** An ingredient in artichoke leaves helps your liver form bile — a juice necessary for good digestion. Too little bile means your food doesn't break down properly, leaving you with bloating, stomach pain, and indigestion after normal-sized meals. Ancient Romans used artichokes to treat indigestion, and they may work for you, too. Small artichokes make great appetizers, and larger ones can be stuffed with a variety of fillings and served as an entrée.

2 **Banish a cough with bananas.** You don't have to take cough syrup. Bananas can calm a chronic cough. A cough that just won't quit combined with a burning sensation in your throat after meals could signal heartburn and acid reflux. In fact, one in 10 chronic coughers can blame heartburn for their troubles. Bananas may bring relief. Try eating one when indigestion rears its fiery head, and see if it helps your cough as well. You can also try banana powder — a dried, ground form of the fruit sold in health food stores.

3 **Serve a side of brown rice.** Add a side of hearty brown rice to any dish that usually causes heartburn. Whole-grain foods like this one help soak up excess acid. Besides nixing heartburn, you could also lower your chances of getting an ulcer. Harvard research suggests that eating lots of high-fiber foods cuts your risk of ulcers. The insoluble fiber in brown rice is the kind that could help the most.

TIP Cooking

Brown rice needs no rinsing. Unlike white rice, it still has its outer bran layer, so it doesn't have sticky starch on the outside. Save time, effort, and water — skip the rinse.

4 **Toss a "bitter" salad.** Try a secret known by dogs — "bitter" greens ease an upset stomach. Dogs eat grass to soothe bellyaches and aid digestion. You can do the same. Instead of grass, nibble on salad made with watercress, endive, and dandelion greens. These herbs stimulate the flow of digestive juices, a boon for older adults and other people who don't produce enough stomach acid. So sit down to a side of bitter greens with dinner. Grate an orange peel on top to add more digestive boost.

5 **Settle your stomach with ginger.** Some spices are considered "bitters," too — like ginger. This rhizome increases the flow of saliva and gastric juices, speeding up digestion and stimulating appetite. This spice also eases heartburn, indigestion, bloating, and gas. Slice chunks of ginger and toss them in a stir-fry or salad, or make a delicious, after-meal tea. Simmer three to four slices of fresh ginger root in two cups of water for 10 to 15 minutes. Go easy at first. Add ginger to your diet a little at a time so it doesn't irritate your mouth or stomach.

6 **Pull the plug on gas with peppermint.** A hot cup of peppermint tea could be just the thing to soothe bloating, gas, and indigestion after meals. This herb stimulates the flow of bile, helping break down fats and squashing gas and bloating. It also encourages you to burp, relieving built-up air in the stomach, plus eases indigestion. Simply pour a cup of boiling water over 1 to 2 tablespoons of peppermint leaves, and let it steep for 5 to10 minutes. Drink it between meals, up to four cups a day.

Watch out!

Tasty tummy tamers they may be, but peppermint and spearmint can actually aggravate heartburn in some people. Peppermint, in particular, seems to relax the lower ring muscle of your esophagus, allowing acid to wash up from your stomach. You may want to avoid peppermint- or spearmint-flavored teas and chewing gums if you tend to suffer from heartburn.

7 **Savor the flavor of cinnamon.** Strike at both gas and indigestion with one super spice. Cinnamon contains essential oils known as volatile oils that help break down fats and trigger movement along your digestive tract. Try it yourself by using a cinnamon stick to stir your next cup of coffee or tea. Or make a tea out of cinnamon. Add one-half to three-quarters teaspoon of powdered cinnamon to one cup of boiling water. You can drink up to three cups a day of this special spicy brew, but never eat cinnamon oil. It's toxic even in small amounts.

8 **Dig into yogurt.** If dairy products give you gas, you may be lactose intolerant. The lactase enzyme, normally found in the small intestine, helps break down lactose, a sugar in milk and other dairy foods. Some people don't make enough lactase, and that problem can worsen with age. Without this enzyme, your body cannot completely digest dairy, leading to gas and other problems. You can still get your calcium by switching to yogurt. Lactose-intolerant people can often digest yogurt easier than other dairy foods because the bacteria in yogurt break down some of the lactose in advance. Check the label. *L. acidophilus* bacteria predigest lactose, but two other kinds — *Lactobacillus bulgaricus* and *Streptococcus thermophilus* — may do an even better job.

Soothe stomach without harming bones

Avoiding dairy doesn't have to mean missing out on calcium if you are lactose intolerant. Canned salmon with edible bones, raw broccoli, oranges, and pinto beans are all good sources of this important mineral. Also, look for foods with added calcium. Fortified orange juice, for instance, has almost as much calcium as milk.

210

9 **Quell gas with caraway.** Herbalists know caraway as a stomachic, a medicine that stimulates the actions of your stomach. In particular, caraway seeds can help cut down gas caused by cabbage. So the next time you stew up a favorite cabbage dish, sprinkle in some caraway for extra flavor. Or brew a spot of caraway tea by crushing one to two teaspoons of seeds, then steeping them in two-thirds cup of hot water for 10 to 15 minutes.

10 **Chew fennel to crush gas.** The seeds from this aromatic herb are a well-known ingredient in spices, soups, and stews — and for good reason. Fennel seeds and greens contain a compound called terpenoid anethole, which can help relieve muscle spasms in your stomach and intestines. Fennel also encourages the production of bile. Together, more bile and fewer spasms can spell relief for gas, heartburn, indigestion, and stomachaches. Chewing the seeds or brewing them into a tea releases these special anetholes. Steep a teaspoon of fennel seeds in one cup of boiled water for 10 to 15 minutes, then strain and enjoy. Crush the seeds first for a stronger flavor.

TIP
Buying

Fresh is best when it comes to fennel. You can grow the herb at home, or buy the seeds fresh at natural food or health food stores. Fennel seeds in the grocery store are probably too old to treat stomach troubles.

11 **Chew gum to end heartburn.** When heartburn heats up your stomach, reach for a simple stick of chewing gum. Scientists say the act of chewing stimulates the flow of saliva, which contains natural antacids. This extra spit neutralizes acid in your esophagus and washes it back into the stomach. One recent clinical trial showed that chewing gum for an hour lowered acid levels in the esophagus of people with gastroesophageal reflux disease (GERD) for three hours. Chew a stick after meals or whenever heartburn sets in. Most people should stick with sugar-free gum to prevent cavities, but some people get gas, bloating, or diarrhea from artificial sweeteners like sorbitol. If you're one of them, stick with regular gum.

Common heartburn culprits	
Plant foods	**Others**
tomatoes	caffeine
grapefruit	alcohol
radishes	tobacco
oranges	carbonated drinks
peppers	spicy foods
onions	greasy, fatty foods
garlic	chocolate
spearmint	mustard
peppermint	vinegar

12 **Douse the fire with water.** One of the best ways to douse the fire of acid reflux comes right from the tap. Water washes acid out of your esophagus and down into your stomach where it belongs. Plus it dilutes the acid in your stomach to help prevent heartburn in the first place.

Drink a glass of water an hour before meals and an hour after. Avoid drinking it with meals when you need the acid to digest food. Sip it throughout the day, too, in small amounts. Drinking too much at once can distend your stomach and actually lead to heartburn. If your problem is indigestion, carbonated water is the better choice, according to one European study. Participants who drank about 1.5 quarts of sparkling water a day saw both their indigestion and constipation get better.

13 **Pile your plate with pears.** Snacking on high-fiber fruits like the Asian pear can help you beat heartburn. One recent study linked a high-fiber diet to a lower risk of heartburn and GERD symptoms. For one thing, eating foods high in fiber and complex carbohydrates such as fruits, vegetables, and whole grains speeds up digestion. Your stomach empties faster, so you have fewer episodes of heartburn. Fiber also fends off constipation. "One of the things that worsens heartburn is any degree of constipation. Treating constipation sometimes — not always — can alleviate or reduce heartburn," says Dr. Timothy C. Wang, chief of the Division of Gastroenterology at the University of Massachusetts Medical School. Asian pears fit the bill. One large pear packs a whopping 9.9 grams of fiber.

Fiber Adequate Intake (AI)

Men over 50 – 30 grams/day

Women over 50 – 21 grams/day

14 **Crunch cauliflower to cool heartburn.** High-fiber diets may protect you from GERD, but high-fat diets put you at risk. Out of 371 people in one study, those who ate the most saturated fat, total fat, and cholesterol were most likely to suffer from GERD. And the more saturated fat and cholesterol a person ate, the worse their symptoms. That makes sense, since fat triggers a chemical change that relaxes the lower esophageal sphincter (LES), the valve between your stomach and esophagus that seals out stomach acid. When it relaxes at the wrong time, acid washes up into your esophagus. Fatty foods also cause your stomach to empty slower, so food and acid stick around longer. Substitute low-fat vegetables like cauliflower, spinach, and asparagus for fried sides at mealtime.

TIP
Storing

Wrap celery in aluminum foil as soon as you get home, and it will keep for weeks. Or place it in a paper bag with the outside stalks and leaves on it for best storage. If it still goes limp, perk it up fast. Trim the ends, and soak it in water up to half an hour. Don't use hot water — only water that is tepid or downright cold will do the trick. Your celery will regain its snap in no time flat.

15 Snack on celery to cut calories.
Eating fewer calories is definitely a tried-and-true weight-loss strategy, but it may also help control heartburn. European researchers tested a low-fat, high-calorie meal versus a low-calorie meal. Those eating fewer calories suffered fewer episodes of acid reflux over the next four hours. The low-calorie food appeared to decrease stomach acid and empty out of the stomach faster. In the process, the LES, the one-way valve between your stomach and esophagus, closed up faster. Cutting back on daily calories could be worth trying. The next time you need to munch, turn to celery. A stalk of raw celery contains only six calories. An ounce of regular potato chips, on the other hand, packs 155 calories. Serve a

vegetable tray with low-fat dip instead of chips at your next party, and enjoy the event heartburn-free.

16 **Fight fire with fiery peppers.** Hot chili peppers may not be the first thing you think of eating when your stomach gives you trouble, but maybe they should be. Chili peppers are healthy for the same reason they're spicy — a compound known as capsaicin. The active ingredient in peppers, it increases blood flow to the stomach, encourages digestive enzymes to start working, and kills the bacteria that produce gas. These actions cut down on gas, bloating, and nausea after meals. Capsaicin also overwhelms the nerve endings in your stomach, limiting their ability to communicate pain, plus puts a lid on the amount of substance P in your stomach — the brain chemical that carries pain signals. This blocks the feeling of pain in your gut. If you're new to hot peppers, start with small amounts, and gradually add more as you get used to them.

Watch out!

Hold the peppers if you suffer from ulcers or chronic heartburn. They can irritate your stomach. Even people without these ills can get indigestion from hot peppers. So know your limits when it comes to spicy foods.

A Closer Look
Recognizing – and avoiding – GI problems

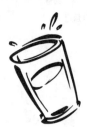

G.I. Joe may have been your childhood hero, but later in life your focus shifts to another GI — your gastrointestinal tract. Your GI tract, which runs from your mouth to your anus, can be the site of many health problems, from constipation to Crohn's disease. And not even G.I. Joe can save you from these GI woes. However, smart nutrition and healthy habits can. Watch out for the following conditions that can affect your gastrointestinal tract — and take steps to overcome them.

Irritable bowel syndrome (IBS). These muscle spasms in the stomach or intestines are known as spastic colon, nervous bowel, or simply IBS. The cause remains unknown, but stress and depression can aggravate it. It isn't life-threatening, but it can affect your quality of life.

Inflammatory bowel disease (IBD). Inflammatory bowel disease, which is much more serious than IBS, includes Crohn's disease and colitis. Your intestines will show evidence of an actual disease process, and your doctor will likely prescribe medicine. Symptoms of ulcerative colitis may include rectal pain and cramping, bloody diarrhea, stomach area pain on the left side of your body, nausea and appetite loss, and fever. Although you may have fever with Crohn's disease, you may also have unexplained weight loss, painful spasms in your stomach area, and intermittent diarrhea.

Constipation. Consider yourself constipated when you have infrequent or hard to pass bowel movements.

Diarrhea. Diarrhea is the opposite of constipation. It's marked by the urgent need to relieve yourself, and loose, watery stools at least three times in a day. Diarrhea often comes with cramps and abdominal pain, bloating, nausea, and fever.

Nausea. This uneasy feeling in your stomach sometimes leads to vomiting, which ejects your stomach's contents through your mouth. You might experience fever, sweats, weakness, unnatural paleness, abdominal cramps, and dry heaves.

Heartburn and indigestion. Indigestion simply means poor digestion. Acid indigestion, or heartburn, occurs when your stomach contents back up into your esophagus, the tube that carries food down your throat. Symptoms include burning in your chest or throat and chest pain, especially after eating or lying down. You may also have a sour taste in your mouth, bad breath, a lump in your throat, difficulty swallowing, chronic hoarseness, sore threat, wheezing, or night cough. Belching, nausea, and vomiting may also occur. Frequent heartburn can be a symptom of gastro-esophageal reflux disease (GERD).

Lactose intolerance. When you're lactose intolerant, you have trouble digesting milk and other dairy products. This happens when your small intestine doesn't produce enough of the special enzyme that breaks down lactose, the main sugar in dairy foods. Symptoms include nausea, cramps, diarrhea, bloating, and gas.

Hemorrhoids. These painful, itching masses form inside your rectum or on the surface of your anus. What's more, they can bleed. Report any bleeding to your doctor because it could indicate a more serious condition, like colon cancer.

Celiac disease. Celiac disease, also called celiac sprue, causes the hair-like villi of the small intestine to become inflamed and flattened. And since nutrients from food are absorbed through these tiny villi, the disease often leads to symptoms of malnutrition — even if you are eating healthy meals. The culprit in celiac disease is gluten, a protein found in wheat, barley, rye, and oats. Symptoms include weakness, anemia, bone pain, weight loss, stomach bloating, and diarrhea or bulky stools that float.

Ulcers. These sores in the lining of your stomach or the beginning of your small intestine may bring on weight loss, poor appetite, burping or bloating, and nausea or vomiting. Gnawing stomach pain comes and goes for days or weeks at a time, occurs two to three hours after meals or in the middle of the night, and goes away when you eat or take an antacid. Most ulcers are caused by a bacterium called *Helicobacter pylori*, or *H. pylori*.

Diverticular disease. Diverticula are pouches that develop in the weakened walls of the intestine. These pouches can become inflamed and infected from bacteria in bits of food that get trapped there. You may experience fever and severe pain, usually in the lower left abdomen. It can also cause gas, constipation, diarrhea, and blood in your stool.

For all these conditions, it's best to pinpoint the foods that trigger flare-ups, and avoid them. You may have to adjust your diet in other ways — such as eating smaller meals — to avoid aggravating your symptoms. Focus on getting more fiber, too — it helps speed waste through your digestive tract and softens your stools. However, you may need to limit fiber with some diseases, such as IBD.

Good nutrition is critical to a healthy digestive tract. Talk with your health care provider about your best course of action if you suffer from any of these conditions.

Bowel disease basics

18 foods to cure intestinal ills

According to Greek myth, a king called Tantalus angered the gods so much that they sentenced him to forever stand beneath delicious fruit he could never reach.

People with inflammatory bowel disease (IBD) or celiac disease can understand what that's like. Some are afraid to eat because they may trigger diarrhea or other miserable symptoms. Others eat, but cannot absorb important nutrients through their damaged intestines. Deficiencies often accompany these conditions, so always check with your doctor in case you need supplements to avoid a health emergency.

Next, discover the incredible power of natural nutritional strategies, and learn about your disorder. The more you know, the better you can manage your condition.

Inflammation in the intestines is at the root of these disorders. Ulcerative colitis involves inflammation of the colon and rectum, while Crohn's disease can pop up anywhere in your entire digestive tract. In people with celiac disease, or celiac sprue, gluten from foods flattens and inflames the hair-like villi of the small intestine.

The cure for celiac disease is a zero-gluten diet. Crohn's has no cure but you can learn to live with it. Although surgery that removes the colon also removes ulcerative colitis, many avoid this drastic surgery and just manage their symptoms through diet and lifestyle. So can you.

1 **Comfort your gut with cooked rice.** Crohn's has sky-rocketed in Japan as fiber consumption has dropped, a Japanese scientist reports. His research suggests the rise of Crohn's may be linked to a plunge in rice intake. Perhaps people need the resistant starch in rice. This starch is so tough that it withstands stomach acid and reaches the bowel undigested. This encourages the growth of probiotics, valuable bacteria that naturally occur in your colon and help defend it. Bacteria and resistant starch are also a recipe for butyrate, a compound that may pro-tect against inflammation and IBD in your colon.

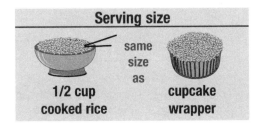

Serving size

1/2 cup
cooked rice

same
size
as

cupcake
wrapper

2 **Feel your oats.** Resistant starch helps your body make the most butyrate, but soluble fiber — like the kind in oats — can help you make some, too. Soluble fiber dissolves in water, forming a gel that slows food down in your intestines. That's what gives your body the chance to make butyrate. And if you're worried about whether you can toler-ate oats, try rolled oats. They're the easiest to digest — plus they're scrumptious with blueberries, another soluble fiber source. If you can't eat oats at all, try psyllium. Research sug-gests it may help prevent symptom flare-ups of ulcerative colitis and also help ease diarrhea in both kinds of IBD.

3 **Eat yogurt and pack in probiotic power.** Yogurt — or its probiotics — can help both IBD and celiac disease. Just six weeks on the probiotic supplement VSL#3 helped 77 percent of people with mild or moderate ulcerative colitis improve, according to a new study. In other research, peo-ple with Crohn's disease cut their risk of symptom flare-ups by taking Mutaflor, another probiotic supplement. The bacteria that ferment yogurt are also probiotics. Experts say you need up to 10 billion of these bacteria daily — about what you'll find in a cup of yogurt. Besides, if you have the lactose intolerance that's common in people with IBD and celiac disease, yogurt is an easier calcium source to digest than milk. Just be sure to check the label for "active cultures" before you buy. If you'd also like to try probiotic supplements, talk to your doctor first.

4 **"Iron" out this short-age with lentils.** About one half of all adults with celiac disease have iron-deficiency anemia. Iron deficiency is also more likely in people with IBD due to blood loss from inflammation of the colon. Iron supplements can cause bowel irritation and cramping, and they can be dangerous if you take too much. So ask your doctor whether you need iron supplements to treat anemia or whether you should rely on food instead. Lentils can be a great source of iron and long-lasting energy, especially for those with celiac disease. Try them in homemade soup or all by themselves. On the other hand, if the risk of IBD symptoms means you're afraid to try lentils, beans, and other high-fiber foods, consider low-fiber, iron-rich foods like clams or chicken.

Eat to control IBD

▸ Cut back on red meat and alcohol. New research shows that diets high in these may triple the risk of ulcerative colitis relapse.

▸ Be wary of high-fiber foods that can lead to cramps and diarrhea.

▸ Eat five to six small meals instead of three large ones.

▸ Try a low-fat diet. High-fat foods may cause cramping and diarrhea.

▸ Eliminate various spicy foods, like hot peppers, until you learn which ones mean trouble.

▸ Avoid dairy if it triggers symptoms, or use lactase enzyme caplets.

5 **Beat magnesium deficiency with artichokes.** Both IBD and celiac disease can hinder your ability to absorb magnesium. If you're not already getting the recommended daily amount, artichokes can help you get there. Try steaming them until they're tender, and dip them in light mayonnaise blended with lemon juice or plain yogurt mixed with Dijon mustard. Add more magnesium to your diet with green peas, potatoes, sweet potatoes, molasses, spinach, okra, scallops, or beans.

Magnesium DRI

Men — 420 mg

Women — 320 mg

6 **Bite into butterhead to cut losses.** Switch from iceberg lettuce to delectable butterhead lettuce, and you'll get four times as much vitamin K. And you may need it badly because celiac disease, drugs for IBD, or ongoing diarrhea can raise your odds of being deficient in this vitamin. In fact, if you bruise easily, have excessive bleeding, or have nosebleeds, you may already be running low. Getting more of this vitamin will help your blood clot properly and may help you evade anemia and osteoporosis. Start by adding butterhead lettuce — sometimes labeled as Bibb or Boston — to your next salad. It has a smidgen of fat to help your body absorb vitamin K. Talk to your doctor about vitamin K if you're on a blood thinner like warfarin or if you're considering supplements.

7 **Drink fortified orange juice.** People who have IBD or celiac disease often absorb less vitamin D than average, and researchers suspect they also may have a higher risk of osteoporosis. Adding more vitamin D could help prevent brittle bones as well as keep muscles strong. One way to get it is through fortified orange juice, so read the labels until you find one that fits the bill. Making fortified o.j. a part of your morning breakfast will give your bones a good start every day.

8 **Dodge disaster with sports drinks.** Diarrhea from Crohn's, colitis, and celiac disease can leave you dehydrated — meaning you're not only short on water, but electrolytes, too. Electrolytes are salts and minerals — such as potassium, sodium, calcium, and magnesium — normally found in your blood, tissue fluids, and cells. Loss of electrolytes can cause serious problems. Although sports drinks can help rehydrate you and restore electrolytes, save them for symptom flare-ups because they have more sugar and salt than you really need. If you're out of sports drinks, diluted fruit juice will do. Use two parts water to one part fruit juice.

Fend off dehydration

This home remedy is simple and quick to make. Sip it to help avoid dehydration from diarrhea.

3/4 teaspoon table salt

1 teaspoon baking soda

4 tablespoons sugar

1 cup orange juice

4 cups water

9 **Win two ways with turkey.** High-fat foods can cause cramping and diarrhea. One way to cut the fat is to choose turkey over other types of luncheon meat. It's usually lower in fat. In addition, turkey can add zinc to your diet. You're probably losing this mineral if you take steroids for IBD — and you need zinc's wound-healing power.

10 **Resist rising risk with chickpeas.** Not only do people with IBD have a higher-than-average risk of colon cancer, but if you take the drugs sulfasalazine or cholestyramine, you're probably also losing folate — a B vitamin that can help control colon cancer risk. Ask your doctor whether you need a supplement. Meanwhile, add more folate-rich chickpeas to your diet. If you can't tolerate high-fiber foods, try low-fiber folate sources like raw spinach or canned condensed chicken noodle soup.

Don't drink the (well) water

A new study from Belgium suggests that drinking well water may be linked to a higher risk of Crohn's disease. How is that possible? Some researchers have suggested that Crohn's may come from the same microbe as Johne's disease, a cattle disease with similar symptoms. Johne's disease is caused by a bacterium called *Mycobacterium avium paratuberculosis* (MAP). MAP may sneak into lakes and streams near herds — a possible express route into local water supplies, such as wells.

11 **Pounce on pumpkin protection.**
Just a half cup of canned pumpkin can deliver as much vitamin A as a whole cup of raw carrots. And that's good news because vitamin A may help protect the lining of your intestines. Besides, people with celiac disease and those taking medicine for IBD symptoms are more likely to be deficient in this vitamin. Try puréeing pumpkin into soup for a year-round treat that puts more vitamin A in your day.

12 **Fight back with potassium-rich lima beans.** This is one food you can rely on when prescription steroids drain potassium from your body. Buy limas frozen for the most flavor, and rinse them to remove the added salt. Potassium deficiency can cause confusion, weakness, drowsiness, dizziness, kidney damage, paralysis, irregular heartbeat, and, sometimes, death. So make potassium-rich foods a priority. You'll also find this mineral in leafy greens, cantaloupe, oranges, potatoes, whole grains, and bananas.

13 **Make it marinara for mighty antioxidants.** Research suggests that people with IBD may have lower levels of antioxidants than normal. Getting more vitamin E may help you fight back. Both marinara sauce and olive oil deliver vitamin E, and your body may absorb the vitamin better when it's in liquid form. So the next time you crave Italian food, try rice or pasta topped with marinara sauce and a little olive oil.

14 **Get more vitamin C from cranberry juice cocktail.** It could have even more than orange juice made from concentrate if you choose products with the most cranberry juice and least sugar. Some experts believe people with Crohn's could benefit from higher amounts of antioxidant vitamins such as vitamins E and C. And, in a recent study, vitamin C was part of a six-ingredient nutritional supplement that helped reduce the minimum steroid dosage needed to control ulcerative colitis symptoms.

15 **Discover collard greens for milk-free calcium.** At least one study suggests that many with IBD may avoid dairy products — and their calcium — due to lactose intolerance. But recent research has experts worried that people with IBD may also have a higher risk of osteoporosis. The good news is that leafy greens like collard greens, kale, and turnip greens can help you add calcium without milk's consequences. You'll be glad you did because your damaged intestines may absorb calcium poorly, and some

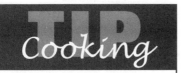

Cooking

Here's a calcium builder for anyone who has lactose intolerance with IBD. Save your shrimp shells, and store them in the freezer. Find a good shrimp stock recipe that starts with shells, and you'll have a high-calcium stock you can use in soups, sauces, and more.

drugs prescribed for IBD steal calcium from your body. You can shred and steam collards and other greens and add them to soup during the last minutes of cooking.

16 **Get big nutrition from a small pack of sardines.** Getting the nutrients you need can be tough when you have IBD. Fortunately, canned sardines not only give you calcium, vitamin D, and omega-3 fish oils, but also selenium. Studies suggest that people with IBD have low blood levels of selenium, so you probably need more. Besides, selenium may help lower the increased colon cancer risk that comes with IBD. And if you're worried about mercury in fish, you'll be glad to know smaller fish — like sardines — accumulate less mercury. But don't just eat sardines and other seafood. Enjoy Brazil nuts, chicken, turkey, and enriched white rice for even more selenium.

17 **Throw symptoms out with rainbow trout.** Scientists already knew supplements of omega-3 fish oils could help prevent relapses of Crohn's disease. But an exciting new study suggests that a supplement with omega-3 oil has helped people with ulcerative colitis. Those who took the supplement for six months needed fewer steroids to control their symptoms. These oils are the same omega-3 fish oils you'll find in delicious rainbow trout. Just remember to limit your consumption to 12 ounces or less per week because some fish may contain mercury or PCBs. Fish oil supplements are usually contaminant-free, but they can also have side effects. Talk to your doctor about how much fish to eat and whether omega-3 supplements are right for you.

18 Uncover the potential of pineapple.

Two older adults improved their ulcerative colitis symptoms with bromelain supplements, according to a medical report. In fact, an endoscopy of one of them even showed that her intestine walls had healed. Of course, supplements have more bromelain than fruit, and it's too early to tell whether fruit-based bromelain can lead to the same symptom-fighting results. But if you can tolerate pineapple, why not enjoy more of this nutritious fruit to find out what it might do for you? Just remember to buy it fresh. Cooked and canned pineapple are used for gelatin dishes because neither has enough bromelain to prevent gelatin from setting. But if you're eating pineapple for health benefits, fresh is better.

Safe foods for celiac disease

You'll find tons of information about gluten-laced foods people with celiac disease can't have. But here are some examples of the foods you can eat.

▶ yogurt, aged cheeses like cheddar and swiss, sour cream

▶ dried peas and beans, lentils, white potatoes, sweet potatoes

▶ all plain fruits and fruit juices

▶ breads, bread products, and cereals made from rice, corn, soy, potato, and bean flour, or from arrowroot, corn, or potato starch

▶ rice, rice noodles, and any gluten-free item made from tapioca, cornmeal, buckwheat, millet, flax, sorghum, amaranth, and quinoa

Ulcer rescue

17 foods to quench the fire in your belly

Avoid stress and spicy food. At one time, that was the only prescription doctors could give you for gastritis and ulcers. Positive action to cure or prevent ulcers was pretty much unknown until the mid-1980s. That's when scientists discovered almost all ulcers are caused by a bacterium called *Helicobacter pylori*. This corkscrew-shaped bug burrows through a protective mucous coating and infects your gastrointestinal lining. Digestive juices follow, and the small sore becomes an ulcer.

Controlling gastric acid may ease the pain and burning of an ulcer, but it won't usually go away until you kill the *H. pylori*. The scientists who made this amazing discovery won the 2005 Nobel Prize for medicine.

Gastritis is an inflammation of your stomach lining, also caused by *H. pylori*, which leads to ulcers. Peptic ulcers can be either gastric (stomach) or duodenal (upper intestine) and can lead to bleeding ulcers, cancer, and other severe conditions. Other things can cause ulcers, but *H. pylori* is responsible for 90 percent of all duodenal ulcers and up to 80 percent of gastric ulcers.

About half of all humans have *H. pylori*, and 10 to 15 percent of those will develop ulcers. Doctors use antibiotics and acid reduction drugs to get rid of ulcers, but overuse of either of these medicines can create other problems.

Today you can take positive steps to control *H. pylori* before it produces the burning abdominal pain of ulcers. Make these simple diet choices to keep the fire out of your belly.

1 **Banish bacteria with broccoli sprouts.** Johns Hopkins University scientists have discovered a special phyto-chemical in baby broccoli that can wipe out *Helicobacter pylori* better than any other natural compound and, in some cases, better than antibiotic drugs. The "magic ingredient" is sulforaphane, and broccoli sprouts contain 20 to 50 times more of it than regular broccoli. You can find broccoli sprouts in supermarkets and health food stores. Use them in soups, salads, and sandwiches, or as a garnish on main dishes. Sulforaphane apparently acts like a natural antibiotic with the ability to destroy *H. pylori* in hard-to-reach areas of your stomach lining. It also knocks out strains resistant to regular antibiotics.

2 **Rely on cabbage for ulcer protection.**
Cabbage has long been a folk remedy for ulcers. It is the head of the brassica family, well known for improving digestive health and preventing cancer. The secret is cabbage's ability to kill *H. pylori* and protect your stomach lining with weapons like sulforaphane, vitamin C, beta carotene, lutein, and glutamine. It's also high in fiber and low in fat and calories — a perfect health food. You can fix cabbage in a variety of ways. Chop it up and make slaw, or add it to other salads. You can boil it, cook it with corned beef, or let it ferment into sauerkraut or kimchi.

Cabbage cocktail cure

Raw cabbage juice is an old home remedy for ulcers. A quart of cabbage juice a day, in divided doses, for 10 days is supposed to make you feel as good as new. Some say it's the amino acid glutamine in cabbage that does it. Glutamine is a favorite fuel for the cells in your stomach lining and may help heal damage done by an ulcer. See your doctor first, though. Ulcers can be dangerous if left untreated.

3 **Put a different spin on spinach.** Since childhood you've heard why spinach is good for you — stories about iron, eyesight, and Popeye's muscles. But did you know spinach also helps your stomach? This poster child for leafy green vegetables is full of carotenoids, and research proves the more carotenoids in your system, the lower your risk of gastritis and other stomach problems. Another study discovered that eating spinach and cabbage lowers your risk of stomach cancer, which — like gastritis and ulcers — is connected to *H. pylori* bacteria. Spinach is also strong on ulcer fighters vitamin A and fiber.

Crucifer or brassica?

Cabbage, cauliflower, broccoli, and brussels sprouts belong to the botanical genus *Brassica*, the Latin word for cabbage. *Brassica* is just one of hundreds of genera in the family *Brassicaceae*, which was formerly called *Cruciferae*, because their flowers often have four petals that look like a Greek cross or crucifix. That's why they're sometimes called crucifers or cruciferous plants. The International Code of Botanical Nomenclature still allows the name *Cruciferae*, even though it's officially changed to *Brassicaceae*.

4 **Choose cauliflower.** It has all the same nutrients that help the other crucifers protect your stomach lining from *H. pylori*. But many people view its creamy-white florets as more elegant than other members of the cabbage family. Mark Twain even described cauliflower as "cabbage with a college education." Cook cauliflower until just slightly tender to lock in important nutrients and cut down on its strong cabbage-like odor.

5 **Turn on to turnips.** The turnip belongs to several food groups. First, it's a species of brassica so it has the same ulcer-fighting qualities as its broccoli and cabbage cousins. It is also a greens plant like spinach, kale, collards, and mustard. And it's a root vegetable like beets and carrots. Except for carrots, roots generally are not as nutritious as their leaves, so your gastric system gets more protection from turnip tops than from the turnip itself. Try sautéing blanched turnip greens with chopped onion and minced garlic in a little olive oil until tender. Cooked turnips can be boiled, roasted, mashed, or diced and added as a flavoring in soups. Thin slices of baby turnips are also good on raw vegetable platters.

6 Pick peppers for vitamin C. This queen of antioxidants is an invaluable weapon in the fight against ulcer-causing *Helicobacter pylori* bacteria. A study of more than 6,000 adults reported that people with low levels of vitamin C were more likely to become infected with *H. pylori*. Those with high levels had 11 percent less chance of infection. Not only does vitamin C kill the bacteria, it also sweeps away toxic byproducts while it boosts your immune system. The best way to get these triple benefits is to eat foods high in vitamin C. Sweet red peppers rank near the top of that list, and they have less acid than the citrus fruits you usually think of for vitamin C. In fact, a third of a raw red pepper has more vitamin C than an orange.

Barley tea stops ulcers

Folk healers say a barley tea can rebuild your stomach lining and cure your ulcer. Cook 2 ounces of pearled barley in 6 cups of water until half the water boils away. Strain and drink the remaining liquid as a tea. Flavor the tea with lemon or honey and eat the barley separately. This same mixture may also cure diarrhea.

7 **Bite into brussels sprouts.** Brassica vegetables are loaded with phytochemicals that fight *H. pylori* bacteria. Among the brassicas, only broccoli has more vitamin C than brussels sprouts. A Tufts University study says these little cabbages may have more total antioxidants than nearly all other vegetables. When you buy different-sized brussels sprouts, cook them in slices so they will all be done before they lose their appealing green color.

Watch out!

After surgery for a peptic ulcer or stomach cancer, your body doesn't produce as much stomach acid. This can be a problem in breaking down certain fruits and vegetables, like brussels sprouts. On rare occasions, an impacted food mass called a phytobezoar will block your bowels and have to be surgically removed. If you think you may be low on digestive juices, go easy on high-fiber foods, and be sure to chew them well.

8 **Cut up a cantaloupe.** A cup of cantaloupe has well over half the vitamin C you need for a day. And it gets its brilliant orange color from beta carotene, which your body turns into vitamin A, another vitamin that helps keep away ulcers. The same cup of cantaloupe gives you twice your daily requirement of vitamin A. Serve this luscious fruit for breakfast, as a snack, or in fruit salad.

9 **Include carrots in your diet.** The Harvard School of Public Health says seven servings of fruits and vegetables every day will cut your chances of developing ulcers. It particularly recommends carrots and other fiber-rich foods. Carrots may be best known for their vitamin A and its positive effect on your eyes, but vitamin A is also an ulcer fighter. It seems to increase the protective mucus in your stomach and intestines. Carrots are good either cooked or raw and can be a handy, portable snack, a fancy side dish, or part of a nutritious salad.

10 **Substitute sweet potatoes for white potatoes.** You'll get the most vitamin A in colorful fruits and vegetables, which puts sweet potatoes right up there with cantaloupe and carrots. This tasty tuber, from the morning glory family, is loaded with vitamins and minerals and has few calories, virtually no fat, and no cholesterol. It has more personality than plain old spuds and is full of fiber, which is not only good for your digestive health, but also helps rebuild your stomach lining. You get as much or more fiber from a sweet potato as you do from oatmeal, bran muffins, or popcorn.

11 **Opt for onions' antioxidants.**
Onions — one of the best-selling vegetables in the world — are exceptionally rich in anthocyanins and flavanols. These are antioxidants that give them their unique flavor and fragrance. They control gastric ulcers by scavenging for harmful free radicals and may even help stop the spread of *H. pylori* bacteria. They may also prevent the growth of cancer

TIP Kitchen

Get rid of that onion smell by rubbing your hands with white vinegar before and after you chop it. If you don't like the vinegar smell, try using the end of a stalk of celery or a cut lemon instead.

cells in your stomach. The antioxidant quercetin also flourishes in apples and tea, but your body absorbs it much better from onions. This vegetable is an important part of almost every culture because it enhances the flavor of so many foods. It is tough, easily stored, and can be enjoyed either cooked or raw.

12 **Cut caffeine with green tea.** All the extra caffeine in coffee and colas may not give you an ulcer, but it can certainly irritate the one you already have. Green tea has less caffeine than coffee or black tea, so it's a more soothing drink than the others. And if you don't have an ulcer, you'll benefit from green tea's powerful antioxidants, called polyphenols, along with its B vitamins and vitamin C. Experts think it may help prevent a host of conditions, including cancer and heart disease. Give green tea a try if you haven't already. It's about as healthy a beverage as you can find.

TIP

Serving

Use olive oil instead of butter on your garlic bread, and you'll give ulcers a one-two punch. Polyunsaturated fats like those in olive oil prevent *H. pylori* growth in the laboratory, and garlic is a proven bacteria killer.

13 **Crush cloves of garlic.** That releases allicin, a natural compound that acts like an antibiotic while giving garlic its flavor and aroma. Allicin seems to kill almost everything — molds, bacteria, viruses, yeasts, and other parasites. In the laboratory, garlic extracts appeared to slow the growth of four different kinds of *Helicobacter pylori*, the bacteria that causes ulcers. So the next time you cook Italian, Greek, or anything

Mediterranean — remember to throw in an extra clove or two of garlic.

14 **Spread honey on bread.** Eat it an hour before meals and at bedtime to avoid ulcers. Honey's antibacterial powers will help wipe out the *H. pylori* bacteria in your stomach that cause gastritis and ulcers. Just make sure it's unprocessed honey because heat processing destroys its bacteria-fighting enzymes. This natural sweetener also will coat your stomach to ease upset stomach symptoms and shield you from ulcer-causing irritants like alcohol and nonsteroidal anti-inflammatory drugs (NSAIDs). Plus, this jack-of-all-trades helps prevent allergic wheezing and sneezing and heals scrapes and burns.

Popular painkillers cause ulcers, too

H. pylori is not the only cause of ulcers and gastritis. Nonsteroidal anti-inflammatory drugs (NSAIDs), like aspirin and ibuprofen, block enzymes that help protect your gastric lining against digestive juices. You're four times more likely to get an ulcer if you use NSAIDS regularly — especially a stomach ulcer. About one in 10 patients taking low-dose aspirin develop ulcers. If you take NSAIDs frequently, talk to your doctor about alternative medications.

15 **Mind the milk myth.** Long ago, people thought milk and other dairy foods coated the stomach lining and soothed the pain of ulcers. Today we know that's not really true. Modern research has found that drinking milk — or eating any kind of food — does have a buffering effect that can temporarily relieve the pain of ulcers. But then it stimulates new acid production that actually makes your ulcers hurt even more in a few hours. If you don't have an ulcer, milk may make it more difficult for *H. pylori* to get a foothold in your stomach lining. It's also a good source of ulcer-fighting vitamin A. But if you already suffer from the burning pain of gastritis and ulcers, go easy on the white stuff.

16 **Drink cranberry juice daily.** Cranberries and cranberry juice may prevent ulcers the same way they stop urinary tract infections — by getting rid of harmful bacteria. Flavonoids in these little red berries keep *H. pylori* from hanging onto your stomach lining. So a glass of cranberry juice a day may be enough to flush the bugs right out of your system. To get the most from this remedy, make sure you buy 100-percent pure juice.

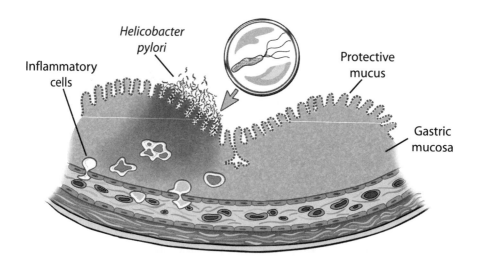

Helicobacter pylori bacteria cause gastritis and ulcers by burrowing into your gastric lining and triggering inflammation. This attack allows digestive acids to burn through the lining, causing a sore.

17 **Add good bacteria from yogurt.** Although their main purpose is to ferment milk into a creamy custard, these bacteria do even more once inside your body. They crowd out bad germs and help your stomach settle all sorts of irritable bowel issues. Researchers have found that certain bacteria may also destroy the *H. pylori* bacteria that cause gastritis and ulcers. If you're being treated with antibiotics, yogurt can help another way. While the medicine kills *H. pylori*, it may also wipe out good bacteria and cause unpleasant side effects, including diarrhea. Yogurt replenishes those good bacteria and also helps prevent side effects. You can get the recommended 10 billion good bacteria per day from just one cup of yogurt with live active cultures.

A Closer Look
Ins and outs of eating out

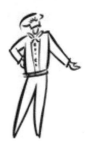

Waiters and waitresses aren't the only ones who could use some tips. Eating out can be a hazard to your health and your waistline if you don't follow these guidelines.

Terrific table tactics

When you were young, perhaps your parents encouraged you to clean your plate. But chances are your plate didn't contain nearly as much food as most restaurants serve today. There's no shame in leaving some food — and some calories — on your plate. One portion-control strategy is to ask for a doggie bag when you order, and put half your entrée in it before you start eating. That way, you won't overeat, and you'll have lunch for tomorrow. You can also split an entrée with a friend.

Consider going out for lunch instead of dinner. Lunch portions tend to be smaller — and cheaper. Another way to get smaller, cheaper portions is to order a few appetizers, rather than a full meal.

Avoid all-you-can-eat buffets. It's not a deal if you save money, but load up on extra calories. If you do find yourself in an all-you-can-eat setting, limit yourself to two trips. Fill a dinner plate with fruits, salads, and other low-calorie vegetable dishes. Use a small salad plate for your second visit.

Sidestep menu mishaps

Before you enter a restaurant, check the menu for healthy choices. If you can't find any, go to another place. Once you've found a restaurant, remember these tips.

- **Avoid fried foods.** They are usually fried in hydrogenated shortening that's bad for your arteries and waistline.

- **Look for dishes with fruits and vegetables.** Chinese restaurants are one of your best bets.

- **Make requests.** Don't be afraid to special order your meal. You're paying for it, after all. Ask to substitute a side order of vegetables for French fries. Or have them bake your food instead of frying it.

- **Ask for sauces and salad dressings on the side.** Then use them sparingly.

- **Limit alcohol.** It just adds empty calories. It's also a good idea to choose plain water over soda.

Just because you're eating on the run doesn't mean you have to take shortcuts with your health. Even fast food can be healthy — if you make the right choices.

Forget the burgers and fries. These days you can find healthier options like salads, wraps, or grilled chicken sandwiches. And choose your condiments wisely. Mustard has only 3 calories per teaspoon, while mayonnaise has 19. If you do opt for more traditional fast food, think small. Pass on the "super-sized" or "jumbo" meals.

Have a pizza craving? Choose thin crust pizza and ask for more sauce and less cheese. Select vegetable toppings rather than sausage or pepperoni. And eat only one or two slices.

Wherever you choose to eat, make sure it's clean. Check the silverware, glasses, dishes, tablecloths, and restrooms. Make sure hot food is hot and cold food is cold at any buffet. Watch out for flies or cockroaches, which spread disease.

Guide to healthy ethnic food		
	Pass on	**Order**
Italian	Alfredo, carbonara, parmigiana, stuffed or fried dishes	Primavera, piccata, marinara, grilled, thin crust
Chinese	Crispy, crunchy, sweet and sour, fried dishes	Steamed dishes, or containing words "jum," "kow," and "shu"
Mexican	Nachos, chimichangas, guacamole, taco salad shells	Fajitas, entrées with shredded meat, soft corn tortillas, salsa, rice, black beans
French	Paté, crème, au gratin, fromage, hollandaise, en croute, béarnaise, mousse, foie gras, pastry	Fruit sauces, or poached, roasted, or en papillote dishes
Indian/Thai/Island	Fritters and coconut dishes	Marinated, steamed, stir-fried, tandoori, Tikka, satay dishes

Kidney comfort

15 foods to vanquish urinary distress

You've been to the bathroom so many times you've lost count. Call your doctor if it doesn't let up quickly. That constant "gotta go" feeling can be a sign of kidney stones or a urinary tract infection (UTI).

Kidney stones are crystals that form when chemicals — like calcium oxalate or uric acid — build up in your urine. Tiny stones may cause no symptoms but larger ones may lead to:

▸ stabbing, irregular pain in the back or side

▸ bloody, smelly, cloudy, or burning urine

▸ frequent urge to urinate

▸ fever, chills, or weakness

▸ nausea or vomiting

Men are more prone to kidney stones than women, but women get more urinary tract infections.

These infections occur when bacteria multiply in your urethra, bladder, or kidneys. Anything that interferes with urine flow can contribute to an infection. For example, men over 50 can develop UTIs due to an enlarged prostate.

Although you probably need an antibiotic from your doctor to recover from a UTI, natural nutritional strategies may help you prevent future UTIs — or ease one now.

1 **Water down your risk.** Good news for people prone to kidney stones and urinary infections — drinking extra water could help you fight back. First, Italian research shows water could slash your risk of having a second kidney stone by 50 percent. Plan for between 12 and 16 8-ounce glasses

of water or other fluids per day. This dilutes your urine and sweeps potential stone-causing particles out of your body. What's more, drinking extra water can also help wash out the bacteria behind urinary tract infections. You're probably getting enough water if you have pale-colored urine. If it's dark, drink more.

Stone-free with coffee and tea?

Even though coffee and tea contain oxalates, a study suggests that drinking them can lower your risk of kidney stones because of their diuretic action. The more you go to the bathroom, the less chance kidney stones have to develop. Both caffeinated and decaf coffee lower risk by at least 9 percent. What's more, tea may cut men's kidney stone risk by 14 percent and women's risk by 8 percent. Although most of your liquids should still come from healthier drinks, these can add variety.

2 **Make lemonade to help your kidneys.** Use this recipe — 4 ounces of lemon juice, 2 quarts of water, and very little sweetener. This refreshing beverage may boost your citrate level, and high levels of urinary citrate may lower your risk of calcium-based kidney stones. In fact, lemonade more than doubled the citrate levels of people with low urinary citrate in a small study, but still reduced urinary calcium. Best of all, a single daily glass could be enough. To get more juice from a lemon, take it out of the fridge, run it under warm water, and apply pressure with your palm as you roll it back and forth on the counter.

3 **Snack on pumpkin seeds.** These convenient, magnesium-rich seeds can help you control oxalate levels. Their magnesium helps your body recycle the oxalates to prevent buildup. Moreover, if you're worried about lost nutrients from high heat processing, you can even dry — not roast — your own seeds. Just remove the seeds from the pumpkin, wash them off, and place them on a cookie sheet. Set your oven to warm, and put the pumpkin seeds in for three to four hours. Stir them often to curb scorching.

4 **Serve spuds to spite stones.** Drizzle lemon juice on a plain baked potato for reinforced kidney defense and a surprisingly tantalizing taste. On top of the stone-fighting power of lemon juice, you'll also receive more than a third of the recommended amount of vitamin B6. Because this vitamin helps change stone-spawning oxalate into other substances in your body, getting enough may block stones from forming. What's more, research suggests a B6 deficiency raises your risk of kidney stones. So add other foods high in B6 like bananas, avocados, chickpeas, tuna, chestnuts, turkey, and fortified cereals.

5 **Get ready for a broccoli surprise.** Studies suggest you'll deflate your odds of kidney stones if you eat broccoli and other good sources of calcium. High calcium in your diet keeps you from absorbing dietary oxalate — that key ingredient for oxalate-based stones. Unfortunately, taking calcium as a supplement may actually raise your risk of stones — so stick with food. Enjoy dairy foods and nondairy calcium sources like canned sardines with bones, turnip greens, and kale. Broccoli may be especially good because it delivers the "fab four" of kidney stone prevention — calcium, potassium, magnesium, and vitamin B6. So devour broccoli florets, and chop or shred the stalks into soups, casseroles, or your favorite stir-fry dish.

6 "Squash" your risk. Low potassium raises your risk of forming stones, but winter squashes — like acorn and Hubbard — can rev up your potassium levels. So steam a winter squash to help protect your kidneys. Just seed the squash, fill a pot with an inch of water, and place a basket or metal colander over the water. Drop squash pieces into the colander and cover the pot. Cook over boiling water until tender. Add even more potassium to your diet with foods like baked potatoes, sweet potatoes, cooked limas, chestnuts, or any canned tomato product.

7 Try rice bran to kick kidney stones. Slip rice bran into breakfast cereals, yogurt, or muffin mixes, and you may reap the same exciting benefits as people in a Japanese study. Sixty percent of study participants were shielded from new kidney stones just by adding less than two tablespoons of rice bran to breakfast and supper. And the group, as a whole, formed fewer stones than before the study. Look for rice bran at health food stores. You may even find it at some supermarkets.

Watch out!

Men with a waist measurement over 43 inches have a 48-percent higher chance of kidney stones than men with a "34" waist, a new study suggests. Stone odds go up by 70 percent for women who have gained more than 35 pounds since age 18. Both men and women can slash kidney stone risk by keeping weight below 150 and limiting body mass index and waist size.

8 Turn wine into protection. A daily 8-ounce glass of wine shrinks kidney stone risk by 39 percent for men and 59 percent for women, according to Harvard studies.

However, alcohol contributes to high blood pressure, liver disease, pancreatitis, congestive heart failure, and many more health problems — so if you don't drink, don't start. If you do drink, limit your alcohol to one or two glasses of wine a day.

9 **Add milk for better kidney care.** Drink low-fat milk to get more of the calcium and extra fluids that help you fight painful stones. Dairy protein also appears to control the amount of uric acid circulating in your blood. Just be sure to keep your milk out of sunlight, bright daylight, and bright fluorescent lights so it won't lose light-sensitive nutrients.

10 **Make popcorn a stone-fighting snack.** Air pop plain popcorn at home, and add your favorite delectable spices to replace the absent butter and salt. Toss it all together with a little olive oil, and you've got a low-calorie snack with stone-slamming fiber. Kidney stone sufferers who eat 10 to 15 grams of bran fiber per day have fewer stones, studies suggest. So have oatmeal for breakfast, two slices of 7-grain bread in a lunch sandwich, a half cup of rice with dinner, and a couple of cups of popcorn for an evening snack. You may shrink your odds of UTIs, too.

Protect your secret

Anyone facing problems with incontinence will be glad to know cranberry juice also works as a urine deodorant. Drink lots of cranberry juice, and your urine will have less of an ammonia odor. So if you have a slight accident, it can be your secret.

11 **Use cranberry juice the wise way.** Don't wait until you get a urinary tract infection to drink cranberry juice. Although dynamic compounds in this juice help sweep out UTI-causing bacteria like *E. coli*, no one has shown it can cure UTIs. But research suggests you can help prevent UTIs by drinking between 8 and 16 ounces of cranberry juice daily. Read product labels before you buy, and look for those with the most juice and least amount of sugar. Sugary sweet drinks may actually help UTI bacteria grow. And when you need a festive break from straight cranberry juice, try this. Freeze some juice in an ice cube tray, and add the cubes to decaffeinated iced tea.

Watch out!

People with a history of oxalate kidney stones as well as those who take the blood-thinning drug warfarin should avoid cranberries. Long-term use of the juice or berries could increase the risk of oxalate stones. And if you take calcium supplements, the oxalates in cranberries can make it tougher for your body to absorb the calcium. Cranberry juice may also increase the effects of warfarin, causing internal bleeding and possibly death.

12 **Discover parsley's purifying power.** Eating fresh parsley will not only give you a vitamin C boost, but it will help you urinate more often. That in turn will sweep out the bacteria that start UTIs. Along with acting as a diuretic, parsley may also freshen your breath after a meal. Why not chew a fresh sprig or two after dining to see whether these benefits work for you? But check with your doctor first if you're taking blood-thinners. The vitamin K in parsley may interfere with these drugs.

13 **Bite into blueberries to blast bacteria.** *E. coli* may be one of the top microbes behind many urinary tract infections, but you could bring it down with blueberries. Their tough antioxidants rough up *E. coli* the way cranberries do — by changing its structure so it can't cling to the lining of your urinary tract. And don't worry about buying too many blueberries. Just eat some now, and freeze the rest for later. Frozen blueberries will keep up to a year.

14 **Eat kiwi and say bye to UTI.** Get friendly with sweet kiwifruits to help make your body hostile to UTI bacteria. Kiwi and other citrus fruits give you lots of vitamin C. Eat them regularly, and you could pick up enough vitamin C to turn your urine more acidic — making it tough for bacteria to grow. You don't even have to peel a kiwi. Just wash it, slice off the ends, cut into quarters, and enjoy.

15 **Add yogurt to reinforce your defenses.** Take a tip from a study in Finland. In addition to your daily cranberry juice, eat yogurt three times each week. Those who did this were less likely to get a UTI, the study reported.

Declare a "no stone" zone

You can help thwart kidney stone formation by following these tips.

▶ Limit dietary fat. Some studies have shown a link between fat and kidney stones.

▶ Limit salt. It steals away stone-stopping calcium.

▶ Cut back on sugary foods.

▶ Avoid grapefruit juice, which inflates risk by up to 44 percent, or apple juice, which raises men's odds by 35 percent.

▶ Check with your doctor before taking calcium supplements or high doses of vitamin C supplements.

Headache healers

17 foods to free you of head pain

Headaches are an occasional nuisance for some people, but for others they are a serious problem. Tension headaches account for about 90 percent of all head pain. You may feel like you have a tight band around your head, causing pain in your forehead and temples or the back of your head and neck.

Less common are cluster headaches, with their sudden, excruciating pain behind one eye. Men get these much more often than women do. Women, however, have nearly three times as many migraines as men. With a migraine, you feel severe pain, usually on one side of your head. Light and sound bother your eyes and ears, and you may feel dizzy and sick to your stomach.

Many things can cause a headache — stress, fatigue, loud noise, bright lights, and hormonal changes. Even skipping meals or eating the wrong foods — especially those containing substances affecting blood flow to your brain — can spell trouble. Some of the most common migraine triggers include red wine, cheese, and chocolate.

Fortunately, many experts believe you can find relief from headache pain just by watching what you eat. Just as some foods can trigger headaches, some foods can help prevent them.

1 **Serve up salmon.** This fish is loaded with omega-3 fatty acids, which help control inflammation. These helpful fats can cut some migraines off before they even start. In a study out of Cincinnati, about 60 percent of the participants had fewer and less-severe migraines after taking fish oil supplements for six weeks. Although fish oil capsules are an easy way to get your omega-3s, it's even better to get them from natural sources like salmon.

2 Mend with mackerel. The omega-3 in this fish will have you saying "holy mackerel!" One reason omega-3 fatty acids help your headaches is because they restore balance between omega-3 and omega-6 fatty acids in your body. Most people get plenty of omega-6 from the common diet. If you don't have enough omega-3, the imbalance causes signals to go off in your brain. Too much signaling triggers inflammation, which leads to problems like headaches. Restore that balance by eating mackerel, a fatty fish full of omega-3.

3 Fix a bowl of brown rice. This dish is known for being rich in lots of different nutrients, but for migraine sufferers, the important mineral is magnesium. People who suffer from migraines typically have lower levels of magnesium than

Herbal headache remedies

▶ **Ginkgo** — This herb helps clear headaches and confusion by increasing blood flow to the brain. The recommended dosage is one 40-mg tablet three times a day.

▶ **Butterbur extract** — Recent research has found that a daily dose of this herb can cut your migraine frequency in half. Look for 75-mg doses at your local supermarket or health food store.

▶ **Feverfew** — This herb has been a valued migraine fighter since 78 A.D. You can chew on fresh, freeze-dried, or heat-dried leaves, or take one 125-mg capsule of feverfew a day.

other people, which makes scientists think magnesium deficiency could be part of the problem. Research seems to back this up. Magnesium supplements helped reduce the number and severity of migraines in one study. But you don't have to take supplements. Making foods like brown rice a regular part of your diet may help you control your headaches.

4 **Pop some popcorn in the microwave.** There is no easier way to get magnesium than to munch on a bag of popcorn. This movie-time snack is a good source of the mineral thought to reduce migraines. An estimated 28 million people in the United States suffer from migraines, and they might be able to prevent them by making sure they get enough of this important mineral.

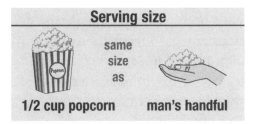

Serving size

same size as

1/2 cup popcorn   man's handful

5 **Make room on your plate for kale.** This leafy green is rich in vitamin B2, or riboflavin. In one study, riboflavin eased migraine pain as effectively as aspirin. Forty-nine people with migraines each took 400 milligrams (mg) of riboflavin a day for three months. Half of them also took 75 mg of aspirin. At the end of the study, 68 percent said they experienced less-severe headaches, whether they took the aspirin or not. Get extra riboflavin in your diet by eating eggs, meat, fish, and green leafy vegetables like kale.

6 **Sauté some mushrooms.** Whether shiitake, portobel- lo, or just the plain old button variety, mushrooms are a gold mine of riboflavin. Get your share of this B vita- min by sautéing some mushrooms in olive oil or chopping them up in a salad.

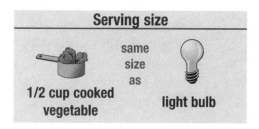

Serving size

same size as

1/2 cup cooked vegetable

light bulb

7 **Always eat your broccoli.** This vegetable is a nutritional powerhouse, but it's the 32 mg of mag- nesium in just one spear that may benefit your headaches. A study of 3,000 migraine sufferers showed that 80 percent of them felt relief from migraines when they took a magnesium supplement every day. Of course, you would have to eat a lot of broccoli to match the 400 mg given in the study. But making magnesium-rich choices each day — including green peas, potatoes, shrimp, and clams — could be enough to head off a headache.

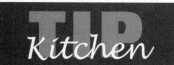

Kitchen

Look for deep green color with maybe a hint of purple when shopping for fresh broccoli. You can refrigerate it for up to four days, but don't wash it until you're ready to cook it. You'll save more nutrients if you steam broccoli rather than boil or microwave it.

8 **Enjoy a bowl of oat- meal.** If you have migraines, melatonin may be the key to relief. Some scientists think migraines may result from an irregularity in the pineal gland located at the base of your brain. This gland produces melatonin, and research has found that migraine sufferers tend to be low in this critical hormone. They are also bothered by environmental factors such as light, noise, temperature, smell, and humidity. Some researchers suggest the pineal gland is the connection between environmental triggers and migraine headaches. Several studies have found melatonin helped relieve pain and prevent a recurrence of migraines in some people. Get more melatonin naturally from foods like oats, which have lots of it. A bowl of oatmeal each morning may be just what you need to stave off that next migraine.

Soothe your headache

The next time you feel a tension headache coming on, try mixing peppermint oil, eucalyptus oil, and rubbing alcohol in a small bowl. With a cotton ball, gently pat the mixture over your forehead and temples, avoiding your eyes. Its cool, relaxing fragrance could be just what you need to feel better.

9 Stir in some wheat germ. Adding this gem of a germ to your oatmeal or cereal will give a good helping of omega-3 fatty acids, a polyunsaturated fat that may help stop inflammation and prevent headaches. You can also mix wheat germ into batter for pancakes, waffles, biscuits, and other breads to effortlessly add this nutritional powerhouse to your diet.

10 Savor the sweetness of sweet corn. This tasty vegetable also happens to be a good source of migraine-relieving melatonin. Researchers conducted a small study using 34 migraine sufferers who experienced two to eight migraines a month. Over three months participants took 3 milligrams of melatonin 30 minutes before bedtime every night. At the end of the study, 25 percent reported suffering no migraines. Another 53 percent saw a

Tension	Migraine	Cluster
mild to moderate pain on both sides of head	moderate to severe pain on one side of head	moderate to severe pain on one side of head
feeling of pressure	throbbing or stabbing feeling	sharp burning or stabbing pain
caused by temporary stress, fatigue, or anger	triggered by food and environment	triggered by food, alcohol, environment, head trauma
muscles around head, face, and neck feel tense	may be preceded by an "aura"	comes on quickly and gets worse fast
no other symptoms	can include nausea, vomiting, sensitivity to light and sound	can include watery eyes, nausea, rapid heartbeat
daily activities still possible	interferes with daily activities	makes daily activities impossible
occurs occasionally and goes away with over-the-counter drugs	occurs often and won't go away with over-the-counter drugs	occurs repeatedly over several weeks

reduction in their headaches of up to 75 percent. Plus, their headaches were less intense and didn't last as long, so they took less medication. You don't have to take supplements to get extra melatonin. A side dish of sweet corn can help, too.

11 **Make life a bowl of cherries.** Cherries are an extra rich source of melatonin, but that's not all they have. Researchers at Michigan State University found that anthocyanins, the same compounds that give cherries their red color, also help squash inflammation. These compounds stop the enzymes that make prostaglandins, hormone-like substances that cause inflammation and pain. Prostaglandins are the bad guys that aggravate conditions like headaches, arthritis, and gout. Eating cherries every day may help relieve those conditions. So give yourself a sweet treat, and eat a handful right before going to bed. They may be just what you need to ward off the nightmare of another migraine.

12 **Ease the pain with ginger.** This spice isn't just for nausea. A woman in Denmark took between 500 and 600 milligrams of powdered ginger at the first sign of a migraine and felt better within a half hour. By making raw ginger part of her daily diet, she ended up with fewer and less severe migraines. Ginger, often taken to ease motion sickness, may also calm the nausea that frequently accompanies migraines. To reap the benefits of ginger, you should eat 1/2 to 1 teaspoon a day. You can eat it raw, steep several slices in a pot of tea, or include powdered ginger in your recipes. But add this spice to your diet gradually. It can cause a burning sensation in your mouth or stomach if you're not used to it.

13 **Stop and smell the apples.** The scent of green apples may do more than make you think of autumn orchards. Studies have found that people who like the smell of green apples reported less severe migraines when they sniffed this scent. Researchers aren't sure why it helps, but aromas can distract and relax you, which may make it easier to handle pain.

14 **Put poultry on the menu.** Our feathered friends turn out to be good sources of the migraine-helping mineral riboflavin. Taking 400 mg of this B vitamin daily could slash the number of migraines you get in half. Get some extra riboflavin into your diet by eating chicken, turkey, and other poultry.

15 **Prevent migraines with fortified milk.** This beverage is rich in both calcium and vitamin D — a combination that may help keep migraines away. Doctors think low levels of these nutrients can bring on these painful headaches. Two women with severe migraines who took large doses of vitamin D and calcium noticed they had dramatically fewer headaches. High doses of vitamin D can be dangerous, but you can get moderate amounts from milk, shrimp, and salmon. Good sources of calcium include milk products, greens, broccoli, and oysters.

16 **Numb clusters with hot peppers.** Capsaicin, the active ingredient in hot peppers, may turn out to be your miracle medicine. In dozens of studies, it numbed pain from common

Hidden headache trigger

A cup of coffee may seem to relieve your morning headache. In fact, caffeine could be the cause of your pain. If your body has come to count on it, missing that drink of cola, tea, or coffee can give you a headache, which then goes away when you drink the caffeinated beverage. The National Headache Foundation recommends limiting yourself to two caffeinated beverages a day. If you drink more than that, cut back gradually. Giving it up all at once could trigger what's called a "rebound" headache.

discomforts, including cluster headaches. The capsaicin causes your body to run out of substance P, the chemical that carries pain messages from your skin's nerves to your brain. Even though the painful condition may still occur, you won't feel it. You can buy capsaicin as a cream, and you must apply it four or five times a day for at least four weeks. It can burn your skin at first, so make sure you use gloves and keep it away from your eyes. But talk to your doctor first if you want to try it for a serious condition like cluster headaches.

17 **Drink a glass of refreshing water.** You may not think a glass of water could cure a headache, but think again. Many headaches are the result of dehydration. The easiest and simplest way to stop dehydration is, of course, to hydrate. Get some water in your system, and that headache just may disappear.

A Closer Look
Hold your food to high standards

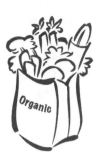

You hear all sorts of advice about which foods you should eat. But what about the quality of the food you buy? How do you know you're getting the freshest, safest food?

Following is a quick guide to food quality, including shopping tips, advice on organic food, the lowdown on mercury and fish, and the dirt on pesticides.

Passing the freshness test

Naturally you want to pay attention to any product's "sell by" date. But there are other things to consider before adding these items to your shopping cart.

▸ **Meat and poultry.** Note the color of meat, which indicates its freshness. Beef should be a bright red, while young veal and pork are grayish-pink, and older veal is a darker pink. When it comes to poultry, look for meaty birds with creamy white to yellow skin. Watch out for bruises, tiny feathers, and torn or dry skin.

▸ **Fish.** A fresh filet or steak will have firm flesh without any gaps in it. If it's fresh, a fish with its head will have bright eyes and red gills. Avoid any fish with patches of slimy or dried-out flesh, blood spots, or other unappealing marks. Fresh fish won't smell fishy either.

▸ **Produce.** Examine fruits or vegetables for firmness and color. Avoid bruised or wilted produce, which may be past its peak.

Organic or conventional?

Organically grown food is more popular then ever — but is it better for you? Studies show no significant differences in flavor, appearance, nutrient content, and bacterial contamination between organic and conventional food. However, organic food contains fewer pesticide residues, and organic meat may be somewhat safer. On the other hand, organic dairy products may not be worth the extra cost.

But there is more than safety and taste at stake. Keep in mind that organic farming is usually more environmentally sound and takes into account social issues — like fair trade and better treatment of labor — as well.

One of the biggest considerations in buying organic is the cost, which tends to be higher than that of conventional products. However, that trend may change as many mainstream grocery stores now offer their own brands of organic food.

It really comes down to personal choice. If you choose to shop for organic foods, federal labeling guidelines make sure you know what you're getting.

- **100 percent organic** — no synthetic pesticides, herbicides, chemical fertilizers, antibiotics, hormones, additives, or preservatives.
- **Organic** — contains 95 percent or more organically produced ingredients.
- **Made with organic ingredients** — at least 70 percent of the product is organic.

If less than 70 percent of the product is organic, the word "organic" can't appear on the front of the package, but it can appear in the list of ingredients.

Minimizing your mercury exposure

Rich in protein and omega-3 fatty acids, fish has long been touted as a healthy food. But recent concern over mercury levels and other pollutants may have you eating like a landlubber. While you shouldn't give up on fish, you should know a little bit about these controversies.

Whether through factories or natural causes, the heavy metal mercury finds its way into bodies of water — and fish. Most people don't eat enough fish to be in serious danger of mercury poisoning, but some people should be careful.

In large amounts, mercury can cause nerve and brain damage. It's especially dangerous for unborn babies and young children because it can hamper their development. That's why the U.S. Food and Drug Administration (FDA) and Environmental Protection Agency (EPA) issued the following recommendations for pregnant women, women who may become pregnant, nursing mothers, and young children.

▸ Do not eat shark, swordfish, king mackerel, or tilefish because they contain high levels of mercury.

▸ Eat up to 12 ounces, or two average meals, a week of a variety of fish and shellfish that are lower in mercury. These include shrimp, canned light tuna, salmon, pollock, and catfish (*see box*).

▸ Check local advisories about the safety of fish caught in local lakes, rivers, and coastal areas.

Another fish controversy involves contaminants called polychlorinated biphenyls (PCBs). One study found that farmed salmon, the kind most commonly sold in supermarkets, had much higher levels of PCBs than wild salmon. But others note that the amount of contaminants depended on where the fish were found — and the levels in both the farmed and wild salmon were within the safety standards of the FDA.

Mercury levels in common seafood

Which fish contain the most mercury? Which have the least? Here are the mean levels of mercury, measured in parts per million (ppm), of some common seafoods.

Fish	Mercury levels (ppm)
tilefish	1.45 ppm
shark	.998 ppm
swordfish	.976 ppm
king mackerel	.730 ppm
orange roughy	.554 ppm
grouper	.465 ppm
tuna (fresh or frozen)	.383 ppm
tuna (canned, albacore)	.353 ppm
lobster	.310 ppm
halibut	.252 ppm
tuna (canned, light)	.118 ppm
cod	.095 ppm
crab	.060 ppm
scallop	.050 ppm
catfish	.049 ppm
herring	.044 ppm
anchovies	.043 ppm
haddock	.031 ppm
sardines	.016 ppm
salmon (fresh or frozen)	.014 ppm

Nonetheless, it might be a good idea to find out more about where your local market gets its fish. And choose fish that are likely to have low levels of contaminants. These include younger and pan fish, rather than old bottom feeders, or trash fish, and top predators.

Pesky pesticides

When you bite into an apple, you know you're getting good nutrients like fiber, magnesium, potassium, and antioxidants. The one thing you may not count on is pesticides. But you can't be sure your produce is 100 percent pesticide-free. Even organically grown produce can contain some pesticide residues.

According to the Environmental Working Group, the most contaminated fruits and vegetables include peaches, strawberries, apples, spinach, nectarines, celery, pears, cherries, potatoes, sweet bell peppers, raspberries, and imported grapes.

Meanwhile, count sweet corn, avocado, pineapples, cauliflower, mangoes, sweet peas, asparagus, onions, broccoli, bananas, kiwifruit, and papaya among the least contaminated.

That doesn't mean you should completely avoid certain fruits or vegetables. So far, there has not been a definitive study showing how pesticide residues affect your health. Just make sure you wash all produce before eating to be on the safe side. Remember, the health benefits of fruits and vegetables far outweigh any potential dangers of pesticides.

Breathing breakthroughs

14 foods to boost your lung power

If you've ever gone even a few seconds without breathing, you know how scary it can be. Shortness of breath isn't something you should ignore. It could mean you have asthma.

This condition occurs when your airways become sensitive and tighten up, making it difficult to breathe. Triggers could be anything from allergens and other airborne irritants to respiratory infections and exertion. With an asthma attack, you may experience coughing, wheezing, shortness of breath, and chest tightness, especially in cold weather or exercise.

More than 25 million Americans — 2 million over age 65 — have had asthma during their lifetime. Contrary to popular belief, many people suffer their first asthma attack after age 70. And, surprisingly, this asthma is often a result of allergies.

Allergies, though not as serious as asthma, are certainly bothersome, and can aggravate an asthmatic condition. You are considered allergic if your immune system overreacts to a normally harmless substance, called an allergen. Common allergens are mold, pollen, dust, and pet dander.

You may not expect food to help you combat allergies or asthma, but certain nutrients can help open up your airways and improve your breathing. If you suffer from these problems, put the following foods on your shopping list.

1 **Eat apples — skins and all.** Apple skins contain lots of quercetin, a specific antioxidant — called a flavonoid — that helps your body fight cell damage. Experts think quercetin helps lower your chances of lung disease, helps keep asthma in check, and may make your lungs work better. A recent study found that quercetin may even help prevent lung cancer. Eat apples — peel and all — five times a week for a punch of antioxidant power and improved lung function.

2 **Get sweet protection from a sweet potato.** Vitamin E is a powerful antioxidant found in sweet potatoes that may cut your risk of asthma. A study in Saudi Arabia found that children who had the least vitamin E in their diets were three times more likely to get asthma. Research also shows that vitamin E helps protect you from developing this condition as an adult. It also protects your lungs from free radical damage, which lowers your risk of cancer. Choose baked sweet potatoes over regular potatoes to reap these healthful benefits.

3 **Fight tobacco exposure with soybeans.** If you lived with a smoker when you were a child, you were exposed to secondhand smoke and probably suffer from respiratory problems in adulthood. You can't turn back the hands of time, but you can load up on dietary fiber. A recent study of 35,000 adult non-smokers in Singapore showed that getting a lot of fiber as an adult can protect against health problems resulting from childhood secondhand smoke. Participants who had lived with a smoker as a child were more than twice as likely to have chronic dry cough as adults. But the ones who ate foods rich in fiber were less likely to suffer from those same negative health effects. Soybeans are a great source of fiber, and most of the study's volunteers included soybeans in their fiber-rich diets. You can do the same.

Watch out!

Watch out for sulfite or sulphur dioxide warnings on packages of dried apricots and other dried fruits if you have asthma. Many dried fruits are preserved with sulfites or treated with sulfur dioxide so they'll keep their color and have a longer shelf life. These preservatives don't affect most people, but some people are allergic or sensitive to sulfites. What's more, the preservatives can trigger a life-threatening allergic reaction in some asthma sufferers. Play it safe and buy the untreated kind, or stick with fresh fruit.

4 **Add a twist of lime to your water.** It's a snappy way to add vitamin C to your diet. Studies have found that vitamin C not only improves asthma symptoms, it helps you avoid the disease altogether. Taking 1 to 2 grams of vitamin C a day helped people with asthma breathe easier in one small study. This could be because vitamin C acts as a natural antihistamine. The antioxidant powers of C may also protect you from other serious respiratory problems. Several studies show extra vitamin C can cut your risk of developing pneumonia by up to 80 percent. And with just 200 mg of vitamin C each day, elderly pneumonia or chronic bronchitis sufferers had fewer symptoms and recovered more easily. Citrus fruits — oranges, grapefruit, lemons, and limes — are all near the top of the list of food sources for vitamin C.

5 **Toss cabbage into your casserole.** Prevent the effects of emphysema by eating cabbage, a vegetable rich in vitamin C. A study that checked the respiratory function of 835 men found that the more vitamin C in their blood the better their lungs functioned. These results back up previous studies showing that vitamin C may protect your lungs from damage and help them work better. Taking in plenty of vitamin C may not reverse the damage of emphysema, but it could slow it down or help keep it from getting worse.

6 **Snack on fresh carrots.** People with chronic obstructive pulmonary disease (COPD), which includes chronic bronchitis, emphysema, and asthma, seem to do better when they get more vitamin A. Participants of one study who took vitamin A supplements for 30 days showed significant improvement in their ability to breathe. In a study done on animals, vitamin A actually reversed some of the lung damage from emphysema. Adding more vitamin A to your diet is a simple way to get the disease-fighting benefits of this important vitamin. To do this, you need to eat foods like carrots that are high in beta carotene, the substance that is converted to vitamin A in your body.

7 **Let honey put a sweet stop to allergies.** Flowers are beautiful to look at, but not if you're allergic

Benefit from breathing country air

You may have guessed that living in the country has its health benefits. Now a recent study from Scotland supports that theory. A survey of 2,600 people revealed that, on average, people who live in rural areas are less likely to have asthma and other respiratory problems like wheezing than people who live in the city. One theory is that people in the country are exposed to more allergens, so their immune systems grow to tolerate more, thereby causing fewer allergic reactions.

Allergy-proof your kitchen

Use these tips to get rid of common triggers and enjoy a more pleasant dining experience.

▸ Clean often to avoid grimy buildup that requires harsh chemical cleansers that trigger your asthma. Use hot soap and water, not irritating detergents.

▸ Wash dishes promptly. Dirty dishes in the sink encourage bacteria and invite cockroaches — a prime asthma trigger. Keep garbage containing food particles outside.

▸ Don't wash with antibacterial soap. Research shows battling a few bacteria will actually stimulate your immune system and protect against allergies and asthma.

▸ Prevent mold by getting rid of moisture sources such as leaky pipes and wet carpet or ceiling tiles. Keep refrigerator drip pans clean and dry.

to them. You may be able to put an end to the sneezing and runny nose you get from pollen by simply eating honey. But not just any kind of honey. Find honey made from local flowers full of local pollen, and it could stop your allergic reaction without drugs or uncomfortable side effects. The pollen itself isn't bad for you, just your body's overreaction to it. If you eat it in small amounts in the honey, it tells your immune system the pollen is not a threat. When you breathe it in later, your body won't reject it, and you won't have the same allergic reaction. See if this strategy works for you. Buy locally collected honey at your nearby farmer's market or health food store, and take one tablespoon each day.

8 **Snack on walnuts.** Mayonnaise, margarine, dressings, and processed foods are all full of omega-6 fatty acids. These can make inflammatory diseases and asthma worse. However, foods with omega-3 fatty acids have the opposite effect. Walnuts are a good source of the omega-3s you need to keep a healthy balance. Sprinkle a few on your salad or hot cereal, or mix them into your recipes for some extra crunch.

9 **Give liver a try.** Maybe you're a fan of liver or maybe you haven't wanted to try it. Now is a good time to start because this dish is a good source of selenium, a mineral that works a lot like vitamin E in your body. Several studies show that asthmatics tend to have low levels of selenium. When a test group of asthmatics took 100 micrograms (mcg) of a selenium supplement, their breathing abilities improved. You can add selenium to your diet naturally by feasting on liver, kidney, and seafood. Just be careful if you have to watch your cholesterol. Organ meats such as liver are especially high in cholesterol.

10 **Ease asthma with magnesium-rich avocados.** This mineral acts like a bronchodilator, opening up your lung's airways so you can breathe better. Magnesium also helps ease the muscle spasms of asthma attacks.

Watch out!

You may be familiar with common food allergies like milk, eggs, fish, and peanuts, but according to a study from Michigan State University, you should add sesame to that list. Researchers reviewing trends over the past 50 years noticed that sesame allergy is becoming a significant problem. Pharmaceutical and cosmetic companies, as well as the baking industry, use sesame oil more than ever. Most cases of sesame allergy involve hives and rashes, but some people develop asthma from the exposure. Pay attention to whether or not your food contains sesame if you think you may be sensitive.

Herbal remedies help you breathe easy

If you prefer herbal remedies to pills, you may be
able to stop allergic reactions and asthma symptoms
with two powerful herbs —
butterbur and ginkgo. A
study of more than 180 people in Switzerland showed
that butterbur extract successfully treated nasal
allergies when compared to
a placebo. The herb
reduced hay fever symp-
toms without causing any
undesirable side effects.
And ginkgo can prevent
bronchospasms, a sudden
narrowing of the main air
passages from the wind-
pipe to the lungs.

An avocado supplies about 15 percent of what you need each day of this vital mineral.

11 **Start seeing red with guava.** Lycopene, the carotenoid that gives foods their pink or red coloring, may pro-tect against asthma, according to a small study. Researchers gave people with exercise-induced asthma 30 milligrams of lycopene each day for one week. At the end of the week, more than half the people showed significant protection against asthma symptoms. It's always best to get your nutrients from foods, and in this case, it could earn you double protec-tion. Many foods that contain lycopene, such as guava, are also high in vitamin C.

12 **Fight infections with garlic.** Antibacterial, antivi-ral, and antifungal. These are the three big healing properties of garlic. For thousands of years, man has used garlic in folk remedies to treat all kinds of ailments. But now, scientists have actually identified chemical properties in garlic that do help you heal. If you're fighting off bronchitis and need some extra help breathing, make a big pot of chicken soup with lots of garlic. It just may do the trick.

13 **Open your airways with a cup of joe.** Start your morning with a fragrant cup of coffee, and you may ease your asthma. Caffeine is chemically related to theophylline, a drug used to treat asthma. When you have an asthma attack, the muscles around your airways tighten up and your passages swell, making it difficult to breathe. Caffeine helps relax your bronchial tubes so your airways stay open. Research shows that caffeine can help improve symptoms for up to four hours.

14 **Drink green tea to suppress allergies.** A tickle, cough, or sneeze could be a reminder you need to brew some tea — green tea. Scientists think a powerful antioxidant in green tea called methylated epigallocatechin gallate (EGCG) may have allergy-fighting properties. EGCG appears to block the IgE receptor, which stops your allergic response to allergens like dust or pollen. EGCG also prevents the release of histamine — the culprit behind runny noses and itchy eyes. Earlier studies have shown that similar compounds in green tea may help relieve allergy symptoms, but EGCG appears to be the most potent. Because boiling water destroys some of the antioxidants in green tea, steep it in water that is hot, not boiling, for about three minutes. Drink it before it gets too cool and the tea turns dark brown — a sign the antioxidants are no longer active.

Folk remedy for allergies

Stuffed up with hay fever or other allergies? Try this time-tested cure. Eat a tablespoon of horseradish mixed with a bit of honey. Both ingredients will kill bacteria, while the horseradish will break up mucus and open up your sinuses.

Cold season survival

18 foods to help you stay out of bed

Few things are more miserable than a cold or flu. Colds are so common that almost everyone catches one sooner or later. And though they may seem similar to the flu, colds last just a few days while the flu — with its aches and fever — is more serious. Older adults and people with heart or lung disease have the highest risk of developing a dangerous case of the flu. It puts 300,000 people in the hospital every year. It can also lead to pneumonia and even death.

But sometimes, your problem isn't cold or flu. If your cold symptoms get worse and last longer than a week, you may have sinusitis. Other symptoms include headaches, painful sinus pressure, sore throat, and yellowish-green nasal discharge.

Your best bet is to see your doctor when you're sick. Antibiotics may help a sinus infection, but not colds and flu. They're both caused by viruses — not bacteria — so antibiotics won't send them packing. But your doctor can determine which medicines will work. Eating the right foods is a good backup. They help boost your immune system so you don't come down with a cold or flu in the first place.

1 **"Soup" up your cold defense.** Your mother's classic cold remedy may be just what the doctor ordered. Even when chicken soup was diluted 200 times, researchers found it still interfered with the substances that trigger colds. Another study suggests chicken soup can reduce inflammation to relieve symptoms. Besides that, the hot liquid moistens and clears your nasal passages and gently soothes a sore throat. And if you feel too miserable to make chicken soup from scratch, don't worry. Scientists report that even store-bought chicken soup can do some good. Best of all, chicken soup is heart-warming "comfort food" that can help you relax and recover.

2 **Sip OJ to sap a cold.** A sweet orange may be loaded with carotenoids, folate, fiber, potassium, and vitamin C, but it still may not be your best defense when you're coming down with a cold. Why? Because you get 25 percent more vitamin C from a cup of orange juice. But make sure it's made from concentrate. When researchers examined different brands of frozen concentrate and ready-to-drink cartons of orange juice, they found that frozen juice mixed with water contained more vitamin C. Research shows that vitamin C cuts down on how long and how seriously you're sick. So load up on additional good sources of vitamin C like guava, sweet red peppers, green peppers, strawberries, grapefruit, lemons, limes, and, of course, oranges.

Watch out!

A serving of milk and cookies could help make your sinuses worse. Milk protein can thicken your mucus and make you produce more of it — just what you don't want. And if mold or fungus is behind your sinus infection, then sugar or alcohol can add to your sinus woes.

3 **Pick a pomegranate, crimp a cold.** You need fluids and vitamin C when you feel a cold coming on. Pomegranates can give you both. Your local supermarket may even offer bottled pomegranate juice for on-the-go convenience. But check the label for vitamin C content. At least one brand of the juice has no C at all. If you can't find a high-C juice, buy a pomegranate instead, and make sure you have drinking straws. At home, soften up the fruit with your palm by rolling it on the counter. Then punch a hole in the top, plunk a straw in, and enjoy the freshest pomegranate juice you can get.

Enjoy the full benefit of pomegranates

Pomegranate nutrients aren't just for colds and flu. Their vitamin C plays an important role in vision, fighting infections and bacteria, maintaining your skin, bone and body growth, reproduction, and normal cell development. Scientists think this vitamin may also fight memory loss, arthritis, respiratory distress syndrome, and more. But pomegranates and pomegranate juice also supply high-impact polyphenols — natural compounds that may battle heart disease. Scientists even suspect that pomegranate fruit extract could also help fight prostate cancer and osteoarthritis. More research is coming, so stay tuned.

4 **Try a honey of a remedy.** This smooth golden liquid has anti-inflammatory powers and antibacterial compounds. A couple of teaspoons of honey might help a scratchy throat, too. Try some alone or in a warm cup of tea.

5 **Fight fire with chili peppers.** You can zap a painful sinus blockage or numb a sore throat with spicy little cayenne or chili peppers. You don't even have to eat them by themselves or in the red-hot raw. In fact, you'd better not unless you're used to it already. Instead, chop small amounts of chili peppers into your favorite recipe, and add more next time if you wish. Just remember to wash your hands carefully afterwards. Getting this pepper in your eyes will burn like — well — fire. Sprinkle cayenne powder on any dish instead to keep the heat off your hands.

6 **Mince garlic to mince colds.** Add garlic to a steaming plate of pasta or a comforting bowl of chicken soup, and you'll get much more than tantalizing flavor. Allicin, one of garlic's powerful — and stinky — compounds kills bacteria and cranks up your immune system. In fact, researchers in a Boston University study claimed garlic works like an antibiotic against *Strep, Staph,* and many strains of flu. It also helps fight infections and may even lower a fever. Experts recommend getting garlic's health benefits by eating one-half to three cloves a day either fresh or briefly heated. Garlic loses its potency if cooked too long. Can't eat garlic? Just try supplements that contain aged garlic extract instead.

Sound the 'all clear' for sinuses

You don't even have to bite into an onion to clear your nose of congestion. Just cut an onion in half, and breathe in as deeply as you can. Your sinuses will start clearing themselves out on the spot, thanks to substances you inhale from the onion fumes.

7 **Drown sinus sorrows and more with water.** Drinking extra water fights colds, flu, and sinus infections because it helps rinse germs out of your body. You'll also stiffen your resistance to infection and help your sinuses drain more easily. Drink as much as you can when you're sick because that's when you need more water and fluids than usual. When you can't stand another plain glass of water, add fruit juice or herbal tea. Just make sure the glass doesn't contain more juice or tea than water.

Pick your favorite throat soother

Gargle with these home remedies twice a day, and your poor scratchy throat will thank you. Just remember not to swallow.

▸ Brew some strong tea. Use it warm or cold.

▸ Mix a half-teaspoon of salt into a cup of warm water.

▸ Add a teaspoon each of salt, baking soda, and sugar to a half glass of warm water.

▸ Dissolve two aspirin tablets in a glass of warm water. Don't substitute acetaminophen or aspirin that's buffered or coated.

8 **Bake up sweet potato protection.** Beta carotene is a fabulous phytonutrient that colors sweet potatoes golden orange. Your body turns this beta carotene into the vitamin A you need to fight off infections and help keep your immune system healthy. Although you can get plenty of beta carotene from pumpkin and carrots, sweet potatoes give you a bonus. A half-cup of mashed sweet potatoes delivers about as much vitamin C as a half cup of broccoli or brussels sprouts.

9 **Keep sinuses clear with black beans.** Black beans contain zinc — a vital nutrient that helps build your immunity and reduce the risk of colds and sinusitis. Zinc also helps change beta carotene to immune-boosting vitamin A. Fortunately, just one cup of black beans supplies women with almost a quarter of their daily recommended zinc. And that same cup contains 17 percent of the zinc men should get. Get more of both beta carotene and zinc from foods like canned vegetable beef soup, Napa cabbage, and cooked spinach.

10 Pit avocado antioxidants against sinus misery. An avocado antioxidant called glutathione may rescue your sinuses. Here's how. Glutathione and other antioxidants dwell in your nasal lining to prevent harmful free radical molecules from causing cell damage. That damage may be partly to blame for sinusitis. But Danish scientists found that people with sinusitis had only half as much glutathione in their mucus as healthy people. So it's possible that boosting your antioxidant levels may help prevent sinusitis. It's certainly worth a try. Get a head start by eating glutathione-rich foods like beef, potatoes, asparagus, and — of course — avocados. Try mashed avocado in place of mayo on your next sandwich.

Easy stuffed nose remedy

People with colds who used saline nose spray three times a day fared no better than those who didn't, a study revealed. But a saline rinse may shorten recovery time from nasal surgery and help fight nasal allergies, research shows. To make a saline rinse, mix a half-teaspoon of table salt with 8 ounces of warm water. Empty it into a bulb syringe, and place the syringe in one nostril. Squeeze the syringe to move the saline solution through your nose. Blow your nose gently. Repeat with the other nostril. Clean the syringe.

11 "Beef" up your defenses. Beef is a good source of both germ-busting zinc and glutathione, but choose it wisely to avoid high amounts of saturated fat. Look for meat clearly labeled as "lean meat" or "extra lean ground beef" by the U.S. Department of Agriculture (USDA). If it's not USDA-labeled, look for the words "select" or "light select" on the label.

12 **Kick coughs with pineapple juice.** The American College of Chest Physicians (ACCP) recently recommended that consumers stop using the most common over-the-counter cough remedies. A review of research suggests they may not work. Yet any remedies containing antihistamines that make you sleepy — like the ones in Chlortrimeton or Benadryl — will help stop coughs. But try this remedy if you have a cough and need to stay awake. Mix 8 ounces of warm pineapple juice and two teaspoons of honey for scrumptious natural relief.

13 **Charge up your immune system with currants.** These black, white, and red berries are bursting with vitamin C, a vitamin famous for its immune-building power. Not only can vitamin C help you get over a cold more quickly, it may also help you recover from more

Watch out!

Antibacterial soap is not your best protection from colds and flu. Viruses cause these infections — not the bacteria that antibacterial soaps fight off. Even worse, using antibacterial soaps too often may help certain bacteria grow stronger and develop a resistance to antibiotics.

serious problems, like pneumonia and bronchitis. Just 200 mg a day — about the amount in half a cup of black currants — may be enough to help symptoms improve. But if these berries taste too tart, try them in jams, juices, sauces, or desserts instead.

Gargle more for fewer colds

It may sound unlikely, but a new study suggests gargling with water several times a day may cut your odds of colds by up to a third. Although more research will determine whether gargling really works, why not give it a try and see if it helps?

14 **Turn to tea for better symptom control.** A piping hot mug of tea is more than just comfort food. Tea contains quercetin, a natural antihistamine. Like commercial antihistamines, quercetin can help control your body's release of the substance that triggers sneezing and coughing. So it might help you feel better. Besides, drinking plenty of warm liquids and plain water can help loosen mucus in your lungs, keep fever down, and help flush germs right out of your body.

15 **Rev up your immune system with chestnuts.** Run low on vitamin B6, and you could weaken your immune defenses. But just 10 fresh chestnuts supplies about a quarter of the daily recommended amount, and you can get them in September before cold and flu season starts. After fresh chestnut season, mix canned puréed chestnuts into soups. And enjoy other good sources of vitamin B6 like canned chickpeas, parboiled white rice, and baked potatoes.

16 **Add wheat flour to your baked goods.** *Sinus Survival* author Dr. Robert S. Ivker recommends a combination of selenium and vitamin E to help prevent allergies and sinusitis. Wheat flour can give you both, so remember that when you make bread or biscuits. Whole-wheat flour has twice as much selenium and 10 times more vitamin E than all-purpose white flour. So use half whole-wheat with half all-purpose or bread flour when you bake. Get more selenium with Brazil nuts, fish, and turkey, and extra vitamin E from sunflower seeds, almonds, and spinach.

Straight talk about herbs

▸ Echinacea studies have yet to prove this herb works against colds. Two studies even suggest it does not.

▸ Eucalyptus vapors can help ease congestion.

▸ Ginger can soothe a sore throat and eliminate mucus. The Chinese have used tea made from fresh ginger root against colds, coughs, and flu.

▸ Ginseng has been found to reduce stress and boost the immune system. A new study suggests that taking ginseng extract every day may mean fewer colds.

17 **Bite into spinach for bonus germ-busters.** Spinach helps you resist colds and flu with the triple threat of vitamins A, C, and E. In fact, more than a third of your dietary reference intake (DRI) of 15 mg of vitamin E awaits you in a cup of frozen, chopped spinach. But if you hate cooked spinach, try a salad of raw spinach leaves, strawberry slices, almonds, and sunflower seeds. Although raw spinach has less vitamin E than cooked spinach, sunflower seeds and almonds have plenty. If you're a woman, a cup of raw spinach meets your daily need for vitamin A and gives you more than 10 percent of your vitamin C. The strawberries will boost the vitamin C even more.

Cold Symptoms	Flu Symptoms
stuffy and/or runny nose	cold symptoms PLUS
sore throat	headache
sneezing	fatigue
coughing	muscle aches
–	fever, chills

18 **Top off your defense with apricots.** In New Orleans, they talk about "lagniappe" — meaning "a little something extra." And that's just what you'll get if you add sunny slices of fresh apricot to oatmeal or fortified cereal — or just snack on dried apricots throughout the day. That will give you a bonus dose of vitamin C and beta carotene, the twin foes of colds, allergies, and infections. And that bit of lagniappe could make you feel a whole lot better.

A Closer Look
Protecting your immune system

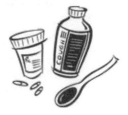

Your immune system is like a sentry on guard 24 hours a day. Or a militia ready to stop any intruder that poses a threat to your health. But who guards the guards? Who protects the protection? You do. That's where a smart diet and healthy lifestyle come in. By knowing how your immune system works and what foods strengthen it, you can help your immune system run at maximum efficiency.

How it works

Trouble can strike your body at any time. Bacteria, viruses, fungi, and parasites attack from the outside, while cancer cells attack from within. Any of these foreign substances, called antigens, stimulate the immune response. Your body counters with its army of white blood cells, including phagocytes, T-cells, and B-cells. They recognize the intruder, mobilize forces, and attack.

For example, T-cells recognize foreign invaders and kill them by breaking them apart. B-cells respond to infection by releasing antibodies, proteins that surround and immobilize the antigens. T-cells and B-cells also have great memories. Once they're exposed to an antigen, they remember it in case it comes back. That's how vaccines work.

Of course, your immune system doesn't always work perfectly. It can overreact to a harmless substance, resulting in an allergic reaction, like hay fever or hives. Sometimes, your immune system can even turn against your own body. That's what happens in autoimmune diseases like rheumatoid arthritis, lupus, and type 1 diabetes.

When you get sick, it's often because the antigen was able to do some damage before your immune system destroyed it. Or because your immune system wasn't strong enough to fight it off.

Diet makes a difference

Your diet has a direct impact on your immune system. In fact, deficiencies of certain nutrients can weaken your ability to fight off disease. To keep your immune system strong, make sure you get plenty of protein, vitamins A, C, and E, omega-3 fatty acids, zinc, selenium, calcium, iron, and antioxidants, including carotenoids like lycopene and beta carotene. These are the building blocks of a strong defense system. Foods that can give your immune system a powerful boost include garlic, onions, and yogurt.

Your best bet is to get these nutrients from foods, not supplements. Talk to your doctor before taking any supplements. If you choose to take them, make sure you buy them from a reputable source.

Beware of fad diets that claim to boost your immune system. They usually involve "cleansing" rituals along with megadoses of vitamins, minerals, and amino acids, which can be unhealthy. Remember, a well-balanced diet will help you build a strong immune system.

Help your body help you

A car needs more than just fuel to run smoothly — it also needs some preventive maintenance. Same with your immune system. Besides eating the right foods, you should also take care of your body in other ways.

▸ **Exercise.** Regular, gentle exercise, like walking, helps fortify your immune system by stimulating natural killer cells that stop viruses and bacteria. Exercise is especially helpful for seniors. Women over 67 who walk or exercise regularly reportedly have fewer respiratory infections than others.

▸ **Get enough sleep.** Your body needs rest to stay in tip-top shape. When it's working to fight off a cold or the flu, sometimes rest is the best medicine.

▸ **Relax.** Find ways to reduce stress, which can weaken your immune system. Listen to music, do yoga or tai chi, go for a walk, practice deep breathing exercises or other relaxation techniques, or just talk to someone about your problems.

▸ **Wash your hands.** It's an easy and effective way to fight germs. When Naval recruits lathered up five times a day, they watched their rate of respiratory illness drop by 45 percent. Wash vigorously with regular soap and water for 15 to 20 seconds.

When you eat right and take care of your body, your immune system will take care of you.

Sleep superstars

13 foods that will send you to dreamland

Ah, a good night's sleep. Just what you need to make your body and brain feel refreshed and energetic. But what if your nights are restless instead of relaxing? Chances are, you feel tired and sluggish during the day.

If you are chronically sleep-deprived, you may have insomnia – the inability to fall asleep and stay asleep. Or a more serious condition called sleep apnea, where you stop breathing hundreds of times a night. You may also suffer from restless legs syndrome – a condition that causes a strange sensation in your legs that makes you need to move them constantly.

If you travel, jet lag could be the source of your woes. In some cases, an illness or a medication may cause your unsettled nights. You need to talk to your doctor if that's the case. Or perhaps it's as simple as having certain habits that keep you awake — like an irregular sleep schedule, too little exercise, or exercising just before bedtime.

Foods can also affect your ability to sleep. Caffeinated coffee and tea can keep you awake, for example, while milk and cherries can help you snooze the night away. Here are some foods you should add to your diet to make bedtime a little easier.

1 **Make a banana smoothie.** It may be the sweet bedtime snack you need to open the door to restful sleep. That's because bananas have melatonin, a hormone that regulates your sleep cycle. Your body is supposed to produce more of it in the evening when it gets dark to help you fall asleep. But some experts believe melatonin production drops as you get older. A good, natural way to boost your level is to snack on foods that contain melatonin — like oats, cherries, tomatoes, sweet corn, and ginger — an hour or so before bedtime. You'll sleep sounder and wake refreshed and ready to face the world when you add these foods to your nighttime diet.

TIP
Serving

Avocados aren't called "butterfruit" for nothing. They make a great substitute for fatty foods like mayonnaise, cheese, sour cream, cream cheese, and butter. Even though avocados are also high in fat, it's heart-healthy monounsaturated fat. Try a slice in place of cheese in a sandwich. Or mash an avocado and spread it on crackers, toast, bagels, or English muffins.

2 Let avocados give you sweet dreams. A restless night robs your brain of what it needs to serve you well throughout the day. But avocados have what it takes to give you back your restful sleep. The hormone melatonin lets you know when it's time to rest, but it can't do it alone. First, your pineal gland converts the amino acid tryptophan into serotonin, assisted by vitamin B6. Serotonin then converts to melatonin. Avocados are a rich source of the vitamin that hurries this process along. A single avocado has 26 percent of the B6 you need each day.

3 Make like a rabbit and eat a carrot. Bugs Bunny's favorite food also happens to be rich in vitamin B6. If you smoke, drink alcohol, have carpal tunnel syndrome, or eat a lot of processed foods, you could run low on this important vitamin. Snack on carrots during the day, or include them as a side dish at dinnertime to replenish your supply of vitamin B6.

4 **Snack on pumpkin seeds.** Experts have found you can use tryptophan and carbohydrates together to tell your body it's time to go to sleep. You'll find tryptophan mostly in animal and fish protein, but you can also get it from pumpkin seeds. If you eat them with carbohydrates, the carbs will aid the release of melatonin. They do this by helping the tryptophan get to your brain through the bloodstream. Once it arrives, your pineal gland converts tryptophan into serotonin and then into melatonin. So the next time you find yourself counting sheep, try snacking on pumpkin seeds with a handful of cereal. The combination will give you just what you need to feel sleepy.

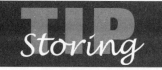

Storing

Cut the leafy tops off carrots before storing. Otherwise, the tops will continue to pull moisture from the carrots, making them dry and bitter. Also, make sure to separate them from fruits that give off ethylene gas, like apples and pears. This gas ripens fruit, but it makes carrots taste bitter.

5 **Sleep soundly with a bowl of barley.** This grain contains melatonin, the natural hormone that helps regulate your internal clock. It's another good choice for a bedtime snack. Eat a bowl of barley soup or cereal an hour or so before retiring for the night. That will

Watch out!

You may be tempted to take a melatonin supplement to help you fall asleep. Don't. Scientists hesitate to recommend it since melatonin supplements are still experimental. Synthetic melatonin has not been tested over the long-term and may cause nasty side effects, including headaches, fatigue, nightmares, and insomnia — the very condition it is supposed to treat. Do yourself a favor, and get your melatonin naturally from foods.

give your body enough time to absorb the melatonin and send you gently off to dreamland.

6 **Eat a handful of cherries.** If you have trouble sleeping, cherries may be your best bet. These little jewels are rich in sleep-inducing melatonin. Although research is still in the early stages, scientists think you may get all the melatonin you need by eating just a handful of cherries a day. A snack just before bedtime would give you the most benefit though. Eating cherries may be especially important if you're older, because as you age, your body doesn't produce as much melatonin on its own.

7 **Enjoy sweet dreams with cheese.** You may have heard the old wives' tale that cheese gives you nightmares, but a study

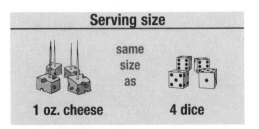

Serving size

1 oz. cheese   same size as   4 dice

from the British Cheese Board claims that is false. The "Cheese and Dreams" study showed that eating cheese before bed could actually help you get a good night's sleep. That's because cheese has tryptophan — the amino acid that helps you make melatonin. None of the 200 volunteers who ate a piece of cheese before bed had nightmares. Almost three-quarters of them slept well every night, and two-thirds also remembered their dreams. Researchers even found that certain cheeses produced certain types of dreams. Hint — if you want to dream about your favorite celebrity, choose cheddar.

8 **Have a bowl of cereal.** Eat cereal or another serving of carbohydrates before bed to help get some Z's. Those carbs will promote relaxation and bring you closer to falling asleep. Choose complex carbohydrates like oatmeal with sliced apples. Grains and fruits break down more slowly than sweet, sugary foods, giving your brain a boost of the feel-good chemical serotonin.

9 **Get to sleep with sunflower seeds.** You've seen bags of sunflower seeds near the checkout counter

Anti-insomnia herbs

No need to count sheep with these herbs. They will help put you to sleep in no time.

▸ **Valerian.** It may work as well as prescription sleep aids without the side effects.

▸ **Chamomile.** It's soothing and relaxing — a great bedtime tea.

▸ **Lavender.** Add five to 10 drops of this essential oil to a steamy bath, or burn a candle made from the oil.

▸ **Lemon balm.** This tasty tea helps to calm your nerves and bring on sweet slumber.

▸ **Marjoram.** Keep this kitchen herb in a bowl on your nightstand to help bring on restful sleep.

in grocery stores. Pick one up next time, and try this popular and healthy snack. It's a good source of both vitamin B3 and vitamin B6, two nutrients that help your body make melatonin. You need a steady supply of these B vitamins to keep your melatonin flowing. Snacking on sunflower seeds is an easy and tasty way to do just that.

Ginkgo gives legs a rest

If leg pain or cramps keep you from sleeping, ginkgo may provide some relief. Many older people have poor circulation in their legs because of hardened or blocked blood vessels. This painful condition is called intermittent claudication. A number of studies show that ginkgo extract relieves the symptoms of intermittent claudication by improving circulation. The usual dosage is 40 mg three times a day, but you probably won't notice a difference for four to six weeks. Check with your doctor to see if ginkgo might help you.

10 Give your body a rest with shellfish.

You probably never thought eating oysters could help you sleep, but the iron in shellfish may help with the effects of a sleep disorder. If you twist your bedcovers into knots with your legs at night, you may have restless legs syndrome. This condition causes creeping, aching, or writhing sensations deep in your legs. The unpleasant sensation only occurs when you're resting and goes away when you move your legs. It is often associated with iron deficiency anemia, so have your doctor check your iron levels. Eating iron-rich foods like shellfish may help. Because too much iron can be harmful, never take supplements without a doctor's advice.

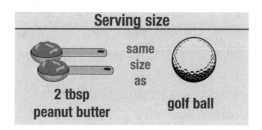

Serving size

2 tbsp peanut butter

same size as

golf ball

11 **Pile on the peanut butter.** Spread peanut butter on whole grain crackers for a healthy snack. Or recapture your childhood and have a peanut butter and jelly sandwich every once in a while. You'll get a good dose of magnesium, a mineral that pitches in to help your body produce sleep-regulating melatonin. A low level of magnesium can result in both insomnia and fatigue. You can get this vital mineral from nuts, green leafy vegetables, and whole grains.

12 **Try dried apricots before bed.** This sweet snack is a good source of niacin, otherwise known as vitamin B3. Niacin also plays an important role in the production of melatonin, a chemical your body needs to help you sleep. Try eating some dried apricots before bed to bring on the Z's.

13 **Drink a glass of warm milk.** This folk remedy has been helping people with insomnia for years. Turns out all those old wives' tales were right. Milk contains tryptophan,

Let a lullabye lull you to sleep

A little night music may be all you need to drift off to the land of Nod. A study from Taiwan revealed that listening to relaxing tunes improved quality of sleep. People between the ages of 60 and 83 experienced longer hours of sleep and functioned better the next day if they listened to soft music at bedtime the night before. Try it yourself. Put on your favorite mellow music, and let those melodies rock you to sleep.

5 ways to conquer insomnia

▸ Go to bed and get up at the same time every day to help set your body clock.

▸ Keep your bedroom dark, quiet, and cool.

▸ Avoid alcohol and caffeine at least six hours before bedtime.

▸ Get regular exercise early in the day.

▸ Relax quietly before bedtime with a warm bath or a good book.

an amino acid that researchers say can help you sleep. It's also high in calcium and magnesium, two minerals that are important in producing melatonin. Another good source of calcium is yogurt, which is easier to digest than milk. And if you haven't already switched to juices fortified with calcium, you should. The juice doesn't taste any different, and cup for cup you'll get at least as much calcium as milk — if not more.

A Closer Look
Adjusting your diet as you age

Age has its privileges — and its pitfalls. Getting older means dealing with several changes, including changes to your body, your lifestyle, and your nutrition needs. Here's how to fine-tune your diet, cope with common problems, and stay healthy in your golden years.

Your changing body

Think of your body as a car. In time, even if you take good care of it, it will start to break down. Or at least not run as smoothly as it once did. Maybe you'll have trouble digesting milk. That's because your small intestine produces less lactase, the enzyme that digests lactose, the sugar found in milk. Try getting your dairy in smaller amounts, which your body should be able to handle. You may also experience increased heartburn, constipation, and other digestive problems.

Your metabolism slows down, and so should your food intake. In fact, you probably need 25 percent fewer calories than you did as a younger adult. But as you get older, your body does not absorb or use some nutrients as well as it used to. This can lead to vitamin or mineral deficiencies. Other nutrients, like calcium, become more important with age (*see box*).

So you have the paradox of needing fewer overall calories but more of certain nutrients. Your best bet is to make your calories count. Limit fats, which have twice as many calories as protein

Don't forget these nutrients

The following nutrients become especially important as you get older. Are you getting enough of them? If not, you may need a supplement.

- protein
- calcium
- vitamin D
- iron
- vitamin C

- vitamin A
- folate
- vitamin B12
- vitamin B6
- zinc

or carbohydrates. Choose foods rich in nutrients and fiber, which aids digestion and soothes constipation. Whole-grain breads and brightly colored fruits and vegetables do the trick. To get enough vitamin B-12 and vitamin D, you may need fortified foods or supplements.

Even if you know which foods you're supposed to eat, you may have trouble chewing them. To overcome this problem, choose easy-to-eat foods that provide the nutrition you need.

- Replace fresh fruit with fruit juices or soft canned fruits, like applesauce, peaches, or pears.
- Substitute vegetable juices and creamed and mashed cooked vegetables for raw vegetables.
- Trade meat for ground meat, eggs, milk, cheese, yogurt, pudding, and cream soups
- Swap sliced bread for cooked cereals, rice, bread pudding, and soft crackers.

Dehydration is also a real concern. As you get older, your thirst mechanism doesn't work as well. But you still need at least 6 to 8 cups of fluid a day. Fluids also help ease constipation. Make an effort to drink more water or other beverages — even if you're not thirsty. (*See box for other high-water choices.*)

Dealing with lifestyle changes

Like your body, your circumstances can change with age. These changes in your personal life often lead to changes in your diet or eating habits.

Perhaps you've lost your spouse and you're adjusting to living alone. The loneliness can make mealtimes unbearable. Cooking may not seem worth the effort, and you may not have much of an appetite. It becomes even more challenging if your spouse normally handled the grocery shopping and cooking. Now you have new skills to learn.

You may be disabled or have problems getting around. Or you could be living on a fixed income, which makes it harder to afford some foods, like meat, poultry, or fish.

Surprising sources of water

Your body needs water — but that doesn't mean drinking it is your only way to get it. Other beverages and even foods can help boost your water intake.

For best results, choose milk, soup, sports drinks, watermelon, strawberries, broccoli, lettuce, and tomato. Other high-water foods include fruit juices, cantaloupe, oranges, apples, pears, grapes, peaches, and gelatin. Peas, frozen yogurt, bananas, eggs, casseroles, and some fish may also help.

Of course, plain old water remains your No. 1 option for staying hydrated. Take a bottle with you, and sip it throughout the day.

No matter what your situation, do not give up on good nutrition. Try these suggestions to make things easier.

- ▸ **Get it delivered.** Check for local programs, like Meals on Wheels, that provide meal delivery or grocery shopping services.

- ▸ **Consider taking cooking classes.** Not only will you learn an important skill, it's also a good way to meet people.

- ▸ **Eat with friends or family.** Or take part in community programs for shared meals with other older adults.

- ▸ **Find other ways to brighten up mealtimes.** Eat with the radio or TV on, for instance. Set the table, like old times.

- ▸ **Keep making nutritious meals for yourself.** Freeze leftovers in single-size portions for days when you don't feel like cooking.

- ▸ **Buy low-cost foods.** Dried beans, peas, rice, and pasta are good choices. Also, clip coupons and keep your eyes open for sales.

Loneliness may not be the only thing affecting your appetite. Ask your doctor if your medications or an illness could be to blame.

Vision defenders

10 foods to keep the world in view

Vision loss doesn't have to be a normal part of aging. Study after study shows that what you eat directly affects the health of your eyes.

Throughout the world, cataracts are the leading cause of blindness. But in the United States, age-related macular degeneration (AMD) takes that dubious honor.

Scientists largely blame ultraviolet (UV) light and oxidative damage for both conditions. Your eyes contain lots of oxygen, polyunsaturated fatty acids (PUFAs), and light-sensitive compounds, all of which are easily damaged by UV light and natural chemical reactions called oxidation.

Luckily, your eyes are also full of protective nutrients — antioxidants, carotenoids, vitamins, and minerals that defend against this damage. You continually have to replenish these nutrients by eating foods rich in them every day. In fact, science is proving that particular foods can slow down or prevent vision loss due to cataracts and AMD.

1 **Cook up kale.** Kale is loaded with lutein and zeaxanthin, two powerful carotenoids that also form the macula, or center, of your eye's retina — the same area that deteriorates in age-related macular degeneration (AMD). Several studies show a link between eating foods high in lutein and zeaxanthin and a lower risk of AMD. These carotenoids protect your eyes from oxidation, a main culprit in macular degeneration. They also absorb harmful blue ultraviolet (UV)

light as it enters your eye, before it damages delicate eye tissue. The same action may ward off cataracts, too. A new lab study showed lutein and zeaxanthin protected eye lens cells from ultraviolet light. In fact, they were almost 10 times more powerful at guarding against UV rays than vitamin E. Aim for 6 milligrams (mg) of lutein per day in your diet. Just a quarter cup of cooked kale or spinach, or a half cup of collards or turnip greens, will do the trick.

2 **Bake a butternut squash.** You can lower your risk of AMD with vision-saving vitamin A. Butternut squash is a grade-A source of the antioxidant beta carotene, a carotenoid your body turns into vitamin A. Antioxidants like this one may safeguard your retina from free radical damage and keep the blood vessels surrounding your eye working properly — all factors that protect against AMD. This nutrient may also cut cataract risk in smokers. Just one cup of this baked squash provides 1,144 micrograms (mcg) of vitamin A, far more than the 700 mcg women need, or the 900 mcg men need each day. Experts say other deep orange or dark green fruits and vegetables like sweet potatoes, carrots, spinach, and broccoli are also unbeatable sources of beta carotene.

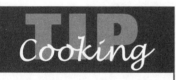
Cooking TIP

Bake butternut squash whole for the most taste. Pierce the rind with a fork several times. Place on a baking sheet, and bake at 375 degrees Fahrenheit until tender. When done, cut it open, take out the seeds, and enjoy the soft, delicious flesh.

3 **Serve a slice of beef.** Your eyes rely on zinc more than you may think. This mineral is heavily concentrated in your retina where it protects delicate vision cells from free radical damage. In the process, it may help defend against macular degeneration. Unfortunately, the amount of zinc in your retina declines with age, and research links low levels of zinc in your blood and in your diet to a higher risk of AMD. Recently, researchers followed the eating habits of more than 4,000 healthy people for eight years.

The benefit of beef

Three ounces of bottom round — the suggested meat serving size — provides around 5 mg of zinc. That puts you well on your way to the recommended 8 mg a day for women and 11 mg for men.

Those who ate foods high in zinc and vitamin E had the least risk of developing AMD. Red meat like beef provides the best source of this mighty mineral, with seafood such as oysters and crab coming in a close second. Your body absorbs zinc best from meat, but barley, black beans, and whole-grain breads leavened with yeast are also good sources.

4 **Keep an eye on almonds.** Cut your risk of cataracts in half by taking advantage of this rich source of vitamin E. Scientists have found that people with low levels of E have a high rate of cataracts, and vice versa, leading them to believe this nutrient may help prevent cataracts from forming. A new study finds that eating high-E foods may also prevent age-related macular degeneration (AMD). Out of more than 4,000 people, the ones who got at least the RDA for vitamin E in their diets lowered their risk of developing AMD. According to this study, researchers say eating foods high in vitamin E is more helpful than taking supplements. Almonds are an excellent source of this valuable vitamin. Just 1 ounce (about 23 nuts) gives you half the 15 milligrams of vitamin E you need every day.

5 **Bring on the broccoli.** Cataracts become more common and more severe as you age, and scientists have linked the problem to lower levels of vitamin C in the lens of your eye. But evidence suggests loading your plate with high-C fruits and vegetables, like broccoli, could lower your risk. Experts say eating more than 300 mg of vitamin C daily for a number of years may cut your risk of cataracts. Believe it or not, broccoli has more vitamin C than an orange, ounce for ounce. In fact, studies specifically link two vegetables — broccoli and spinach — to fewer cataracts. A cup of cooked broccoli with dinner gets you closer to your high-C goals with 101 mg of vitamin C. Toss in some sliced sweet red peppers, add a cup of fresh strawberries for dessert, and you'll have eaten more than 300 mg of vitamin C in just one sitting.

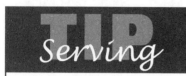

TIP
Serving

Cook vegetables lightly and handle fruits gently to preserve their treasure trove of vitamin C. This nutrient can easily be destroyed by oxygen and heat. For best results, eat fresh fruits and vegetables soon after buying them.

6 **Try an exotic mango.** In all this eye-opening excitement over vegetables, don't forget to eat your fruit, too. Fitting more fruit into your day may stave off future vision problems, including AMD and cataracts. In a study from Harvard University and Brigham and Women's Hospital, researchers examined the eating habits and eye health of more than 77,000 women and over 40,000 men. People who averaged three or more servings of fruit each day dropped their risk of "wet" AMD, the more severe form of the disease, by 36 percent. A new study of nearly 40,000 women found similar results for cataract protection. Those who ate the most fruits and vegetables sliced their cataract risk by 15 percent compared to women who ate the least. So give mangoes a try. They're absolutely bursting with eye-healthy nutrients, like beta carotene, vitamin C, and vitamin E.

7 Feast on fatty fish. Omega-3 is a kind of polyunsaturated fatty acid essential for eye health, and you get it almost exclusively from food. As part of the Nurses Health Study, researchers looked at more than 70,000 women over 16 years. They found that those who ate the most omega-3-rich fish — at least three servings a week — had a 12 percent lower risk of cataracts than women who ate less than one serving of fish a month. Other studies suggest high omega-3 intake from fish may fend off age-related macular degeneration (AMD) as well. People who ate the most fish packed with EHA (eicosapentaenoic acid), a special type of omega-3, were only half as likely to develop advanced AMD as people who ate the least. Research suggests eating as little as one serving of fish each week may raise your protection against AMD. For the most omega-3, feast on fatty fish like salmon.

New!

Two new drugs may actually reverse vision loss from wet AMD, the more serious, less common form of the disease. In wet AMD, blood vessels grow abnormally in the retina and leak blood and fluid into the eye. This slowly leads to vision loss. The new drugs stop these vessels from growing and may restore lost vision with few side effects. One drug, Macugen, is already available. The other, Lucentis, is still being tested as of early 2006, but shows even more promise.

8 **Sprinkle on curry spice.** Turmeric, a spice used in Indian curry dishes, contains a compound known as curcumin. It's an antioxidant that may help fight off cataracts, especially in people with diabetes or hyperglycemia (high blood sugar). In a recent rat study, curcumin and turmeric slowed the growth of diabetes-related cataracts, perhaps by countering some of the oxidative damage caused by hyperglycemia. But be careful. Some curry mixtures contain salt, and high-sodium diets may raise your risk for cataracts. Look for low-sodium curry spices, or make your own (see box).

Add spice, not salt

Make your own salt-free curry blend by mixing:

- 2 tablespoons each turmeric and ground coriander
- 1 tablespoon ground cumin
- 2 teaspoons each ground cardamom, ground ginger, and black pepper
- 1 teaspoon each powdered cloves, cinnamon, and ground nutmeg

Add a dash of it to seafood, poultry, beef, potato soups, salads, and milk-based cream sauces.

9 **Spoon up some yogurt.** Eating foods rich in riboflavin, also known as vitamin B2, may slash your risk of age-related cataracts. Light damages proteins in the eye lens over time, but eating more food high in riboflavin may put a halt to this damage. Two studies found people who got at least 1.6 mg a day of riboflavin from their diet had up to half the risk of cataracts as those who got the least. You may know how valuable yogurt is for calcium and "probiotics," but it is also a good source of riboflavin. Eight ounces of low-fat yogurt gives you about 0.5 mg of this important vitamin. Low-fat milk, spinach, and low-fat cottage cheese are also some of the best, wholesome sources of riboflavin.

10 **Sip wine with dinner.** A glass of red wine may cut your risk of cataracts, according to a new study out of Iceland. In the Reykjavik Eye Study, people who drank moderate amounts of red wine — at least two glasses a month, in this study — had half the risk of cataracts as nondrinkers. Drinking other types of alcohol, including beer and spirits, had little if any protective effect. Men should limit themselves to no more than two drinks a day, and women one drink a day.

Winning smiles

20 foods to help you put your best face forward

Kissing can help you avoid tooth decay and cavities, according to the Academy of General Dentistry. But that's just a good start on a healthy mouth. You can do many other things to help you keep your winning smile.

Bacteria and viruses are your mouth's number one enemies. Bacteria can cause bad breath as well as cavities and gum disease. When bacteria break down leftover food particles in your mouth, they may produce an unpleasant odor. Bacteria can also attach to your teeth, feast on the sugar in your mouth, and leave behind an acid that can cause cavities and gum disease. If your gums are red, swollen, and bleed easily, you may have mild gum disease called gingivitis. This often leads to the more serious periodontitis, a possible first step to infection and tooth loss.

The herpes simplex virus causes fever blisters or cold sores that can be both painful and unattractive. And in a condition called Sjogren's syndrome, your immune system attacks the glands that keep your mouth and eyes moist, causing extreme dryness and discomfort.

A dazzling smile begins with brushing, flossing, and regular dental visits, but what you bite into may also help preserve your grin.

1 **Fend off three ills with yogurt.** This treat can beat up bad breath, defend teeth and gums, and even help block canker sores. In a small study from Japan, six weeks of two yogurts a day reduced the bacteria and chemicals blamed for bad breath. What's more, an 8-ounce container of low-fat plain yogurt brims with one third of the calcium recommended for older adults. That calcium doesn't just keep your teeth strong and healthy. Most gum specialists recommend it, too. You might even prevent canker sores with plain yogurt. Just make sure the label says it contains *Lactobacillus acidophilus,* and eat between four tablespoons and two cups daily. And swish your mouth with water afterward so the yogurt doesn't stay on your teeth. Its lactic acid could undo all the healthy benefits.

2 **Pour more water — prevent more cavities.** In spite of what the dentist says, most of us can't whip out a toothbrush or antibacterial mouthwash after every single snack or meal. But if you drink water when you can't brush, you might avoid the dentist's drill. According to researchers, just rinsing with water could cut mouth bacteria by up to a third. Drinking throughout the day can help, too. So try to get about eight 8-ounce glasses a day.

Kitchen TIP

Make a first-class mouthwash on the cheap. Combine a half-teaspoon salt and a half-teaspoon baking soda with a cup of water for a high-powered weapon against bad breath.

3 **Clip bad breath with cloves.** Not only have cloves long been chewed for fresher breath and toothaches, but dentists also consider clove oil a trusty remedy. You might enjoy clean breath, too, if you brew a few cloves with your tea.

4 **Eat an apple a day to keep the dentist away.** That's right — the dentist. Here's how. Eat crisp apples in place of doughnuts, candy bars, or other packaged snacks, and you'll dodge piles of refined sugar, corn syrup, and other commercial sweeteners. These sugars help plaque build up on your teeth and gums, but naturally sweet apples help you fight plaque. The fiber in apples acts like a scrubbing detergent on your teeth. So if you grab an apple when you can't brush after eating, you may keep your teeth cleaner — and limit your dental visits. When apples aren't available, try celery, carrots, and other fiber-rich foods. They're rugged teeth defenders, too.

Quick breath freshener

Ancient Romans ate parsley to freshen breath, and it may work for you, too. Instead of tossing aside that sprig decorating your plate, save it for a quick after-dinner pick-me-up for your mouth. If you take blood-thinning medication, check with your doctor first before making parsley a regular part of your diet. It's loaded with vitamin K, which can counteract the medicine's effects.

5 **Add buttermilk for fresher breath.** Buttermilk not only dishes up tooth-fortifying calcium but also friendly *lactobacillus* — active "good" bacteria cultures that make it tough for odor-causing bacteria to grow. Drink a little buttermilk to sweeten your breath, or use it as an ingredient in recipes. Try this sour cream substitute for example. Mix three-fourths cup of buttermilk with five tablespoons of melted and cooled butter. Let the mixture set at room temperature for 40 minutes. You'll end up with breath-freshening "sour cream."

6 **Erase cold sores with Swiss cheese.** This famous hole-spangled cheese contains lysine, a powerful amino acid that may erase cold sores more quickly and reduce future outbreaks. Although research has used lysine supplements, you can also get lysine from milk, lean red meat, eggs, fish, lima beans, potatoes, and many cheeses. Just remember that the amino acid arginine can block lysine's benefits, so avoid peanuts, walnuts, seeds, whole grains, rice, and gelatin. Also, find out your cholesterol levels before using lysine. Some studies suggest lysine may push cholesterol up.

Watch out!

Read the ingredients on toothpaste if you're prone to canker sores or cold sores. Studies show that sodium lauryl sulfate (SLS) can be irritating to your poor mouth. Look for toothpastes without this ingredient so you're less likely to raise your risk of sores.

7 **Aim white beans at canker sores.** A six-year case of canker sores was virtually cured in just three months when doctors discovered — and remedied — a zinc deficiency. Scientists have also linked low zinc levels to unhealthy gums. Yet one cup of white beans can deliver close to 3 milligrams of zinc — more than a third of the dietary reference intake (DRI) amount for women and about a quarter of the DRI for men. To prevent gas without soaking the dry packaged beans all night long, add 10 cups of water per pound of beans, and boil for three minutes. Soak one to four hours, and you'll have gas-free beans.

8 **Drink cranberry juice for slick protection.** A new study reports that compounds in cranberries make teeth too slippery for plaque-making bacteria. This may help prevent plaque and tooth decay. Although most commercial cranberry juice cocktails have too much sugar to help fight plaque, unsweetened cranberry juice is available — just hard to find. Check your local health food store for the good stuff. If what you find is too tart, either add water or sweeten it with a tiny amount of natural fruit juice.

New!

Scientists are experimenting with animal and adult human stem cells to grow new teeth — or new tooth material — in animals. If future research continues to be successful, you may someday be able to grow new teeth to replace losses.

9 **Aim for high C with grapefruit.** New research shows that people with periodontal gum disease have low blood levels of vitamin C. But eating grapefruit revs those levels up and may even help your gums improve. If white grapefruit is too sour, try the sweeter red and pink kinds. Just remember that grapefruit can change the way your body handles certain medications — either by blocking absorption or making you absorb the drug faster. Check with your doctor to learn whether grapefruit could affect medicines you take. Meanwhile, enjoy other vitamin C-rich foods like sweet peppers, broccoli, tomato soup, and citrus fruits.

10 **Trample a trio of troubles with milk.** This creamy liquid seems to coat and soothe your mouth when dry mouth is troubling you. It can also help prevent

Watch out!

Studies show that people who get
canker sores and eat a lot of nitrites
are seven times more likely to get cancer of the esophagus.
Nitrites are found in beer, hot dogs, smoked fish, ham, bacon,
sausage, and luncheon meats. But black tea and vitamin C
seem to prevent nitrites from deteriorating into cancer-causing
nitrosamines. So cut back on nitrite-rich foods, and drink iced
tea, lemonade, or orange juice whenever you eat them.

tooth decay. Best of all, cold milk can soothe the pain of eating
with canker sores. Just swish a mouthful around, and swallow
from time to time during your meal. And if you want to pack
more good nutrition into your diet, consider buying organic milk
occasionally. Scientists from the Danish Institute of Agricultural
Research found that organic milk from pasture-fed cows has significantly more antioxidants, omega-3 fatty acids, beta carotene,
and vitamin E.

11 **Give garlic a license to kill.** Garlic can literally be
murder on the bacteria behind gum disease, a
recent British study suggests. Researchers tested
garlic extract containing the compound allicin, a potent
antibiotic that kills a variety of bacteria, viruses, fungi, molds,
yeasts, and parasites. The garlic either inhibited the growth or
killed most of the periodontal organisms tested. You should
probably talk to your doctor before using garlic extract. But
eating garlic may help, too. So break out your favorite Italian
recipes, and give garlic a try.

12 **Fight teeth-harming bacteria with wasabi.**
Wasabi — or Japanese horseradish — is a plant that belongs to the same cruciferous family as broccoli and cabbage. Chemicals in wasabi called isothiocyanates stop bacteria from sticking to your teeth, a study suggests. Try this spicy topping the next time you're at an Oriental restaurant, or buy some to experiment with in your own dishes. You can buy it as powder or paste. Just remember — a little goes a long way.

13 **Beat up bacteria with black tea.** This dark delightful brew kills some cavity-causing bacteria right where they stand. Black tea can also help you wash away other plaque-building microbes before they start making trouble. Just remember to drink your tea plain. Adding milk or sugar just helps the bacteria fight back.

14 **Serve shiitakes to shrink gum pain.** Eat more shiitake mushrooms, and you may stop dreading dental exams. A recent study found that non-smokers who got the most vitamin D were less likely to bleed when examiners probed their gums. Adding more vitamin D may help you fight gum disease, too. Start with dried shiitake mushrooms. Soak them in warm water for one or two hours, and use the reconstituted mushrooms in your favorite soups or stir-fries. Add even more vitamin D to your diet with salmon, fortified milk, or other D-enriched dairy products.

15 **Try raisins to repress cavity-makers.** A promising family of natural raisin compounds could mean a sweet deal for your teeth. According to a new study, these compounds block the growth of bacteria that cause cavities and gum disease. That's surprising because experts previously thought raisins' stickiness contributed to dental decay. On the other hand, the California Raisin Marketing Board funded this study, so independent research is still needed. Yet raisins are a good source of iron, potassium, B vitamins, fiber, boron, and calories. So replace more high-sugar snacks with a sun-mellowed trail mix of raisins, raw sunflower seeds, and nuts. The results may make you smile.

16 **Unleash green tea against gum disease.** Your mouth is under attack, but drinking green tea may help you fight back. One enemy is a nasty little microbe called *P. gingivalis*. It produces toxins that probably promote gum disease and tooth loss. But laboratory studies suggest green tea's powerful polyphenols may hinder the microbe's ability to create toxins and may also fight against the toxins' gum-damaging activities. This fabulous tea seems to battle tooth decay, too. For the healthiest tea, steep it in hot — not

'Health' foods that harm your teeth

You know sweets and sodas can damage your teeth, but some seemingly healthier choices may also erode the tooth enamel that helps protect you from decay.

▸ Canned ice tea and non-cola carbonated drinks. A recent study discovered these types of drinks can permanently harm enamel.

▸ Herbal teas. Another study found that some teas, particularly those with fruit flavorings, might damage your teeth more than orange juice.

▸ Sports drinks, wine, citrus juices, other fruit juices. Their high acidity contributes to dental erosion.

▸ Yogurt. Fermented products contain lactic acid that can harm your teeth over long periods of time.

boiling — water for about three minutes, and drink it without milk or sugar.

17 **Beat that down-in-the-mouth feeling with lentils.** These tiny legumes may be the best-kept secret in the bean world. Their iron and folate can help prevent unhealthy gums and recurring canker sores. Try lentils with enriched rice to pile on even more folate, and you'll also add high-quality protein that is every bit as good as the protein from meats.

Double-cross canker sores

Two remedies are better than one for canker sores. When they first appear, puncture a vitamin E capsule and squeeze the gel directly on the sore. The second remedy — for later use — is a quick fix for canker pain. Just hold a wet tea bag in your mouth over the sore. Keep it there for at least 10 minutes, adjusting the bag for comfort, as needed. The astringent tannins in black tea will help dry up and heal the sore.

18 **Double your defense with sugar-free gum.** You may think chewing gum does your teeth more harm than good. But it can actually have some benefits, provided it's sugar-free. Try chewing sugarless gum for a short while occasionally. You'll increase the saliva you produce, which rinses food particles from your teeth and dilutes the bacterial acid that causes cavities. Sugar-free gum can also help soothe and moisten your mouth if you have dry mouth from medications or Sjogren's syndrome.

19 **Battle B deficiency with this bagel.** Low levels of B vitamins may lead to canker sores, but an egg bagel can help replenish those vitamins. A medium egg bagel supplies more than 45 percent of the DRI for vitamin B1 and around 20 percent of the DRI for vitamin B2. You'll even gain a little vitamin B6. Get more vitamin B1 from foods like enriched white rice, pork, or tropical trail mix. Add vitamin B2 with reduced fat chocolate milk, mushrooms, or fortified cereal. And build up vitamin B6 with chickpeas, an unpeeled plain baked potato, or turkey.

20 **Let honey sweeten your smile.** Honey is so good at killing bacteria and healing infections that doctors use it to treat burns, ulcers, and now tooth decay. A recent study showed that a "honey leather" product chewed for 10 minutes after each meal over a three-week period significantly reduced plaque and gum bleeding. Experts believe honey may work by releasing hydrogen peroxide, a chemical that kills bacteria. Not all types of honey have this power, though. Unprocessed kinds, like you'd find at a health food store, pack the best antibacterial punch.

Skin-saving solutions

18 foods to soften, smooth, and protect

You may not know it, but your skin is your largest organ, and it's the biggest target for harmful free radicals that damage cells and cause wrinkles. This means you have to take extra good care of it. Eating right, especially foods high in antioxidants, will help keep your skin healthy. And don't forget, foods can also be useful on the outside. The ancient Egyptians, for example, slathered honey on their skin to help it stay moist.

Wrinkles and dryness aren't the only threats attacking your outer layers. You can protect your skin from all sorts of problems if you know how. Rosacea is a condition that resembles acne. It's incurable, but you can reduce its effects by shying away from food triggers.

Hives, like rosacea, appear as red patches, but they itch for a while and then eventually go away. They're usually caused by an allergic reaction, so you can find ways to prevent them. Eczema, on the other hand, is a long-term case of itchy skin that pops up especially during periods of stress.

Other skin problems include shingles, body odor, bruises, and burns. The list goes on and on, but the conditions don't have to. The right foods can help give you a fighting chance.

1 **Give yourself an avocado facial.** Your beauty is far deeper than your complexion. But since your skin is such a vital organ, it's important for you to take care of it. Try softening your skin with avocado. It has been used for years as a natural facial treatment, especially for dry skin.

If you suffer from food allergies, you may have to avoid avocados. They're high in amines — tyramine and histamine, in particular. Amines can cause flushing — a common symptom of food allergies and an uncomfortable nuisance, especially if you have rosacea. One remedy — besides avocado abstinence — is to take an antihistamine a couple of hours before eating high-amine foods.

Just remove your makeup and wash your face. Mix some mashed avocado with a little milk or oatmeal, and apply to your face. Let it pamper your skin for 10 minutes, then rinse and enjoy the results.

2 **Rely on a banana beauty tip.** Here's how to save some trips to the beauty shop. For a facial from your kitchen, combine a mashed banana with a tablespoon of honey and a splash of orange juice. Apply to clean skin, and relax for 15 minutes, then rinse off with warm water.

3 **Protect your skin with cantaloupe.** Your skin is more than just pretty packaging. It's a barrier to bacteria that could invade your body. Cantaloupe can play a big role in protecting this barricade because it's loaded with beta carotene. Your body converts beta carotene into vitamin A, which your skin needs to maintain these critical barrier cells. Skin cells that don't get enough vitamin A may be replaced by cells that secrete keratin — the substance that makes your hair and fingernails tough. It also makes your skin dry, hard, and cracked, which increases your chances of infection. Enjoy a bowl of sliced cantaloupe once in a while, and you will reap the benefits of better skin.

4 **Let cauliflower help you avoid bruises.** If you're over 50, you're more likely to bruise. That's because, as you age, your stomach becomes less able to absorb the vitamin K you need to thicken your blood. Eating cauliflower regularly is one way to help solve the problem. A cup of raw cauliflower gives you 16 micrograms of vitamin K — about 18 percent of the daily requirement for women over 50, and 13 percent for men. Cauliflower is a great addition to a party vegetable tray, along with other vitamin K-rich foods like broccoli, carrots, celery, and cucumbers. Just add a little low-fat dressing, and munch to your heart's delight.

TIP

Buying

Get younger looking skin without expensive creams. Scientists from Italy say a compound in lemon juice can protect your skin from the ravages of time. The researchers found that lemon oil protects against free-radical damage, which helps prevent the effects of aging. Look for cosmetic products with lemon oil, but try it on a small area first. Some people may be allergic.

5 **Add more celery to your dishes.** Ultraviolet light can harm skin cells and DNA, causing wrinkles and other damage. Compounds that prevent this damage are called antioxidants. Research has found that eating more antioxidant-rich foods raises the amount of wrinkle-resisting antioxidants in your skin. Fruits and vegetables are famous for their rich hoard of antioxidants. Celery is a good choice, as are leafy greens, spinach, eggplant, asparagus, onions, leeks, and garlic. Try for at least five servings of vegetables, totaling 15 to 17 ounces, each day. If you're not sure how much that is, notice the weight listed on cans or packages of vegetables, and check the scale when you weigh fresh vegetables in the store.

6 **Heal your wounds with honey.** The next time you get a scald or scrape, think of gold — as in golden honey. Just a dab of this homemade remedy will help you heal in several ways. Honey protects your wound while allowing your skin to regrow. At the same time, it reduces swelling and prevents scarring. It doesn't irritate your tissues and is virtually painless to apply and remove. Most importantly, it acts as an antiseptic by slowly releasing bacteria-killing hydrogen peroxide. Almost all ancient civilizations used honey as a treatment for wounds, sores, and skin ulcers, and modern medical studies have supported its healing power. Keep a honey pot in your kitchen, and you'll have a sweetener for your tea — and a handy home remedy.

A honey of a helper

Use honey for more than just burns. Look for this helpful home remedy as an ingredient in moisturizers, body scrubs, bubble baths, and hair conditioners to reap its benefits on a regular basis. Even sun care and sun screen products may have honey in them soon for its moisturizing abilities.

7 **Snack on nuts.** A handful of nuts is a great way to get linoleic acid, a type of omega-6 fatty acid. If you don't have enough of this fatty acid, your skin will become dry, rough, and blotchy. Foods like nuts, wheat germ, and vegetable oils are full of

315

omega-6, but you don't want to go overboard. You need to balance omega-6 with another type of fatty acid — omega-3 — to keep your body at its best.

8 **Enjoy the benefits of water.** Drinking water could be the most important thing you do to help your skin. It moisturizes from within to keep your skin soft and smooth. Here's a tip to help you remember to drink at least six cups a day. Set out six eight-ounce glasses on the counter. As you finish each one, put it in the sink or dishwasher. When you have none left, you'll know you've met your goal. Water can also help relieve the discomfort of rosacea. The next time you feel yourself starting to flush, drink a glass of cold water or chew on ice chips. It will help cool your body temperature and bring down the redness.

Spicy alternatives

Avoid rosacea by swapping these tasty substitutes for spices that trigger redness.

Instead of:	Try:
chili powder	2 tsp cumin and 1 tsp oregano
poultry seasoning	1/2 tsp sage, 1/2 tsp coriander, 1/4 tsp thyme, 1/8 tsp allspice, 1/8 tsp marjoram
curry powder	4 tsp coriander, 2 tsp turmeric, 1 tsp cinnamon, 1 tsp cumin, 1/2 tsp basil or oregano, and 1/2 tsp cardamom

9 **Put on an oatmeal mask.** You've heard of oatmeal facials where people mix water with oats and apply the paste to their faces, and you may have wondered what it's supposed to do. The magic ingredient is beta glucan, a soluble fiber in the cell walls of oat kernels. When you put it on your face, beta glucan penetrates your skin by slipping in between the cells of your skin layer. Oats have been reported to relieve irritation, help wounds heal, and make skin appear smoother. The participants of one study applied beta glucan to their faces and noticed fewer wrinkles in 10 days. Give it a shot, and see if the oatmeal mask works for you, or look for products that include beta glucan in their ingredients.

10 Make fish part of your diet. Many supplements claim to fight psoriasis. One that actually works is fish oil. In several clinical trials, fish oil supplements improved the symptoms of psoriasis, including scales, redness, and itching. Fish has omega-3 fatty acids, which protect your skin and fight inflammation. By making fish a regular part of your diet, you'll reap the benefits of these helpful fats.

Secret to a clear complexion

Folk medicine has used asparagus seeds to treat parasites, toothaches, and hair loss. Although it's not medically proven to work, some people even put a mixture of asparagus shoots and extract on their face to clear up acne.

11 Cook with olive oil. Mixing two tablespoons of olive oil into your daily diet may help your skin. The monounsaturated fats in olive oil resist oxidation and protect your skin from sun damage. Plus, your body needs fat in order to absorb certain antioxidants, so olive oil helps you hang onto protective antioxidants that will reduce wrinkles. Olive oil also has vitamin E, a nutrient that keeps your skin soft and younger looking. Use olive oil or canola oil instead of animal oils or other vegetable oils when you cook.

12 **Sweeten your scent with parsley.** Everybody sweats, but body odor doesn't have to be part of the package. If you want to smell good, your diet can help. Certain vegetables and herbs, like parsley, contain chlorophyll, a natural deodorant that helps prevent body odor.

13 **Pour on tomato sauce.** Lycopene puts the red in tomatoes, but it may also fight disease and tissue damage, according to a small German study. Scientists tested whether lycopene can help your skin overcome the harm caused by sunlight's ultraviolet (UV) radiation. Volunteers ate a dish of tomato paste and olive oil daily for 10 weeks, which gave them 16 mg of lycopene per day. Other volunteers were given olive oil, but no tomato paste or lycopene. Lycopene-eating volunteers showed 40 percent less sunburn than the other volunteers. The lycopene may have helped the skin defend itself against UV damage — and maybe fend off future wrinkles and skin cancer, too.

Try an old-fashioned remedy

A poultice is a warm, thick mixture of herbs, water, and other ingredients that you spread on your skin and cover with a cloth. Try an old-fashioned witch hazel poultice to help dry up an oozing rash and relieve pain. Stir 5 to 10 heaping teaspoons of finely chopped witch hazel leaves into a cup of water. Bring to a boil, and simmer for 5 to 10 minutes, then strain. Press the wet leaves against your rash, and cover the area with a warm cloth to hold it in place.

14 **Have a kiwi for dessert.** Bruises on your body come from broken arteries, veins, and tiny capillaries. Blood seeps under your skin from these

> ## Watch out!
>
> If you take Prozac and occasionally get a skin rash, check your diet. You may be eating too much chocolate. Some folks are sensitive to serotonin, a neurotransmitter that both chocolate and Prozac tell your brain to release. One man in particular broke out in a rash whenever he had a chocolate dessert while he was on the drug. This unusual combination could be causing your woes.

breaks and forms the familiar black and blue mark. If you bruise easily, maybe you're not getting enough vitamin C in your diet. This nutrient strengthens your blood vessels by helping your body make collagen, the protein building block of bones, teeth, blood vessels, and scar tissue. Without collagen to reinforce them, your blood vessels would look like an old, leaky garden hose. To keep your blood vessels strong, eat lots of fruits and vegetables rich in vitamin C, like fresh kiwi.

15 **Learn another reason to love chicken.** It's full of tryptophan, which your body converts into niacin. A deficiency in niacin causes a disease called pellagra, meaning "rough skin." That should tell you how important this B vitamin is for healthy skin. Without it, you can develop the red, rough skin that gives pellagra its name. Plenty of skin-saving niacin can be found in meats, including chicken.

16 **Soothe pain with hot pepper.** Capsaicin skin cream is made from hot red peppers. It may sound strange, but applying the hot pepper cream to your skin actually makes it less sensitive to heat and pain. That's because it gradually deadens the nerves that transmit pain. Research has shown that capsaicin may be effective for several conditions, including arthritis and shingles. With shingles, you should wait until blisters have healed completely before using the cream. Capsaicin products are available as a prescription or over the counter.

Natural skin soothers

For cheap, natural alternatives to those expensive potions, try these solutions to avoid wrinkles and soothe your skin.

▸ Dab some olive oil around your eyes to make crow's feet fly away.

▸ Make an anti-wrinkle mask by mixing 2 tablespoons of honey with 2 teaspoons of milk. Apply to your face for 10 minutes, then rinse and enjoy the results.

▸ Apply the soothing liquid from the leaves of the aloe vera plant to burns, blisters, and rashes to help soothe and heal.

▸ Use almond oil to massage your skin when you need to relax and unwind.

17 **Heal your wound with papaya.** This tropical fruit is a traditional therapy in the Caribbean and Africa, and now modern science praises it, too. A dressing of mashed, unripe papaya removes dead tissue, encourages new skin growth, and reduces infection. It's particularly effective on skin ulcers and burns. If you want to try this remedy, spread a new layer evenly and thickly over your wound every day. Be warned, though, papaya can sting when you first put it on.

18 **Drink tea to bag protection.** Studies show tea acts like a body armor to help shield your skin against harm from the sun's rays. And when you fend off skin cell damage, you may avoid wrinkles and skin cancer as well. Tea is loaded with antioxidants called catechins. These mighty substances neutralize the free radicals that can lead to tissue damage and disease. In fact, some skin care products now contain green tea to help boost your defenses. Whether you get it from a cup or a tube, tea just might help you win the battle against skin cancer.

New!

A new shingles vaccine developed by Merck & Co. may cut your chances of developing shingles in half. It's called Zostavax, and it's basically a stronger version of the children's chicken pox vaccine. Researchers gave the shot to more than 38,000 people over the age of 60. The vaccine not only reduced the number of people who got the condition, it lessened the pain of those who did get it.

A Closer Look
Health claims — facts or frauds?

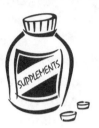

As you browse the supermarket aisles, certain products catch your eye. Maybe the colorful packaging, the brand name, or the low price got your attention.

But what often stands out are the health claims. One product claims it may reduce your risk for heart disease, while another may help prevent cancer. Sounds great, but can you trust them?

It's important to know how health claims work, which claims are approved, and which ones may signal false advertising.

Food label basics

The United States Food and Drug Administration (FDA) strictly regulates the health claims that appear on food labels. Based on solid scientific evidence, health claims link food or nutrients to a reduced risk for a disease or health-related condition (*see box*).

For example, studies have shown that calcium helps prevent osteoporosis. So the label on a calcium-rich dairy product can say calcium may reduce the high risk of osteoporosis in later life. On the other hand, sodium is known to raise blood pressure, so a low-sodium product would toot its horn by saying diets low in sodium may reduce the risk of high blood pressure.

Including these health claims on the label is optional for foods that meet the requirements — but illegal for those that don't.

Recently, the FDA has also allowed qualified health claims when there is emerging evidence to support a food, but not enough for a full-fledged health claim. The wording of these claims is not as forceful as regular health claims and makes it clear the evidence is limited. Some qualified health claims involve green tea and cancer, omega-3 fatty acids and coronary heart disease, and tomatoes or tomato products and certain cancers.

Nutrient content claims — which use words like "free," "low," "reduced," or "good source" — also help you make smart food choices. Like health claims, they are strictly regulated.

But don't believe everything you read. A food can claim to be "fat-free" if it has less than half a gram of fat per serving. That's why pretzels, which actually contain 1 or 2 grams of fat per cup, are considered a fat-free food.

Your best bet is to closely read the Nutrition Facts panel on the label, which contains more detailed information about a food's serving size, calories, and nutrition content.

Shady world of supplements

When it comes to supplements, things get a little trickier. That's because they are not regulated by the FDA. They can still use the FDA-approved health claims, if they meet the requirements. Same with nutrient content claims and qualified health claims.

But many supplement claims fall into the murkier category of structure/function claims. Unlike health claims, structure/function claims can't suggest any link to a reduced risk of disease — just describe how a substance may affect your health. For instance, "echinacea boosts the immune system." Often, research supporting these claims is limited, so it's hard to know what to believe.

Structure/function claims — which can also appear on foods — are supposed to be accurate and truthful, and must include a disclaimer that the claim was not evaluated by the FDA and the product is not intended to "diagnose, treat, cure, or prevent any disease."

Make sure to buy supplements from respectable dealers. Beware of outrageous claims, like "shrinks tumors," or products that claim to be a cure-all for a wide range of problems. Watch out for terms like "scientific breakthrough" or "miracle cure" as well as pressure to act quickly.

Health claims you can count on

The FDA has approved health claims for a number of foods and nutrients, including the following.

Food/nutrient	Condition	Risk
calcium	osteoporosis	lowers
sodium	hypertension	raises
dietary fat	cancer	raises
saturated fat, cholesterol	coronary heart disease	raises
fiber-filled grain products	cancer, heart disease	lowers
fruits and vegetables	cancer, heart disease	lowers
folate	neural tube defects	lowers
sugar alcohol	dental cavities	raises
soy protein	heart disease	lowers
plant sterol/stanol esters	heart disease	lowers
whole-grain foods	certain cancers, heart disease	lowers
potassium	high blood pressure, stroke	lowers

Female focus

16 foods to ease a woman's woes

Being a woman is grand, but it comes with its own concerns, like premenstrual syndrome (PMS), menopause, yeast infections, and fibrocystic breasts. You may never experience PMS, but all women go through menopause and most will get a yeast infection at some point in their lives.

What you eat could help prevent or soothe certain conditions. For instance, foods rich in phytoestrogens may help manage uncomfortable menopausal symptoms like hot flashes, while a daily cup of yogurt could prevent yeast infections.

Food can help balance your mood, reduce hot flashes, slow bone loss, prevent vaginal infections, and reduce cysts in breast tissue. Read on to learn how eating well can help you handle your particular concerns.

1 **Get a lift from little shrimp.** Net some relief from premenstrual syndrome (PMS) with this popular seafood. Shrimp are rich in vitamin B6, a nutrient which helps your body make brain chemicals called neurotransmitters. In particular, B6 helps turn the amino acid tryptophan in foods like turkey into serotonin, a neurotransmitter tied to feelings of calmness and contentment. As a result, this vitamin may improve depression and other symptoms of PMS, including fatigue, breast pain, fluid retention, mood, sleep, and memory. People who smoke, drink alcohol, take estrogen, eat lots of refined foods, or suffer from depression tend to have too little B6 in their bodies. If you're one of them, unwind with a

Hot herb cools hot flashes

The herb black cohosh could help relieve your menopausal symptoms. In a randomized, double-blind clinical trial with more than three hundred women, taking 40 milligrams (mg) a day of black cohosh extract for 12 weeks relieved menopause symptoms, particularly hot flashes, about as well as hormone replacement therapy. Women in the early phases of menopause benefited more than those in the later stages.

healthy cocktail — the shrimp kind — and you may ward off the stress of PMS.

2 **Add almonds to your menopause menu.** Menopause occurs when the ovaries stop producing eggs each month, hormone levels — especially estrogen — drop, and menstruation ends. Half of all women experience it by age 50. Aside from uncomfortable symptoms like hot flashes, the biggest concern of menopause is your drop in estrogen. This hormone keeps a lid on fibrinogen levels — the sticky stuff that helps blood clot. It also lowers "bad" LDL cholesterol while raising the "good" HDL kind. Put it all together, and you have major protection from heart disease. Unfortunately, menopause leaves you newly vulnerable to heart disease. Certain plant foods can help, however. Almonds are rich in phytoestrogens, plant sources of estrogen that offer some of the same protection as human estrogen. So are oats, apples, wheat, and corn. Plus almonds supply calcium needed to thwart osteoporosis, another concern after menopause.

3 **Go shopping for barley.** The phytoestrogens in barley could cool hot flashes among other menopausal symptoms. Plus, barley is full of soluble fiber which can help lower cholesterol and balance blood sugar. Adding it to your diet will help you stay regular and even ward off diseases like colon cancer. Experts don't recommend you eat a specific amount of barley. Just make it and other plant foods like green beans and apples regular parts of your menopausal menu.

4 **Work soy into your diet.** Soy is chock-full of isoflavones, a specific kind of phytoestrogen which seems to ease menopausal symptoms for some women. Asian women often eat a soy-based food like soybeans, tofu, miso, or soy nuts every day, and very few report hot flashes or mood swings during menopause. Isoflavones may deserve the credit. Some research also suggests these compounds decrease bone loss and increase bone strength in older women. Talk to your doctor first about whether soy products could improve your menopause symptoms or bone health — some evidence suggests eating more soy could raise your risk of developing breast cancer or senility.

TIP

Buying

Soy nuts offer one of the simplest, tastiest ways to benefit from the phytoestrogens in soy. These "nuts" are actually whole soybeans soaked in water and baked until they turn brown. High in both isoflavones and protein, soy nuts make a perfect travel snack for munching on the go.

5 **Cool off hot flashes with flaxseed.** This seed contains lignans, a different kind of phytoestrogen. Flaxseed is yet one more plant food that shows promise in reducing menopausal symptoms like hot flashes. A study from the University of Minnesota also suggests it may protect against breast cancer. Plus, flaxseed is jam-packed with fiber which sweeps cancer-causing substances out of your digestive tract before they can do harm, thus slashing your risk of colon cancer. You must crush or grind flaxseed to benefit from its special phytoestrogens. Look for ground flaxseed and flaxseed meal at your local grocery or health food store. You can also buy whole seeds and chew them, or grind them yourself in a coffee grinder and sprinkle atop salads, cereal, and bagels.

Put a stop to hot flashes

Old-fashioned healthy habits may be the safest way to reduce hot flashes during menopause. These lifestyle choices have no harmful side effects and tons of benefits. Relief from hot flashes is just a bonus.

▸ Lose weight.

▸ Quit smoking.

▸ Exercise regularly.

▸ Turn down your thermostat.

▸ Drink cool beverages and eat cold foods.

6 **Grab hold of avocados.** Two of its nutrients make it especially good for you during menopause and beyond. The vitamin E in avocados not only quells hot flashes, it also counters the threat of heart disease that rises dramatically after menopause. As an antioxidant, E protects your arteries from cholesterol damage. Research suggests eating foods loaded with this vitamin can lower postmenopausal women's risk of death from heart disease. The magnesium in avocados helps your body absorb calcium, building your chance at strong bones even as you age. Slice an avocado over salad, or make fresh guacamole for a midday snack.

7 **Eat bok choy to build up bones.** Aside from strengthening bones, some experts think calcium can help treat hot flashes. Whether or not that's true for you, getting plenty of calcium is undeniably important during menopause. In fact, experts recommend menopausal women get 1,200 milligrams of calcium every day. Tired of milk? Vegetables such as bok choy, Chinese mustard greens, and kale come with calcium, too. Chop these greens and add to a soup for a tasty, simple serving of calcium. Eat bok choy raw or lightly cooked for the most of nutrients.

8 **Scramble an egg for strong bones.** However you like them, eggs are rich in vitamin D, otherwise known as the "sunshine vitamin." D is key to building strong bones because it helps your body use calcium. In fact, the American Dietetic Association names vitamin D intake as a leading factor in bone health, muscle strength, and fracture risk. Your body naturally makes vitamin D when you spend time in the sun, but you lose some of that ability as you age. Plus, people who live in northern climates or in smoggy cities may not get enough of the sun's ultraviolet rays to make the amount of D necessary for bone health. Food can come to the rescue. Start your morning off with a boiled egg and a glass of fortified milk for a solid dose of vitamin D. Salmon, shrimp,

Birthday affects age at menopause

Your birthday could affect what age you start menopause, according to scientists in Italy. They interviewed close to 3,000 women and found those born in spring entered menopause at a younger age than those born in autumn. The earliest "bloomers" were women born in March. On average, they began menopause at age 48. Women with October birthdays began it latest, around age 50.

Myths about menopause

Long ago, the ancient Greeks had their own ideas about the source of menopausal symptoms. They believed that menstrual cycles were the female body's way of purifying itself of toxins that built up over the course of each month. When menstruation ended, the Greeks thought those toxins became trapped inside, creating poisonous vapors that rose to the head. These nasty fumes supposedly caused insanity, depression, suicidal thoughts, and general hysteria in menopausal women.

and fortified cereals are other good sources.

9 Pry open a clam to strengthen your bones. Clams are rich in vitamin B12, a nutrient that may help keep your bones strong and prevent osteoporosis. New research links B12 levels with bone mineral density. In a Tufts University study, men with low blood levels of B12 had lower bone density of the hip, while women low on B12 had low bone density of the spine. Researchers think this vitamin affects osteoblasts, a kind of cell that builds and repairs bones. Unfortunately, your body has a harder time absorbing B12 as you age, making it extra important to fit as much as possible into your diet. Clams are hands-down the best source of this nutrient, but you can also get a hefty helping from crab, salmon, trout, and fortified cereal.

10 Make sandwiches with whole-grain bread. Whole-grain wheat, oats, rye, millet, and barley contain a trio of nutrients thought to protect women from recurring yeast infections and chronic vaginitis. Your body naturally harbors yeast in this area, but sometimes it multiplies out of hand. Yeast infections are just one type of vaginitis, or vaginal inflammation. Women with recurring yeast infections are likely to run low on magnesium. Whole grains could help change that. They are less processed so keep more of their original nutrients than refined grains. Enjoy oats or barley for breakfast, and choose pastas and breads that list ingredients such as whole oats, whole wheat, whole rye, cracked wheat, or graham flour first in their ingredient list.

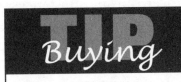

TIP
Buying

Don't be fooled by whole-grain imposters — "wheat flour," "enriched flour," and "degerminated corn meal" are not whole grains.

11 **Spoon up yummy yogurt.** The bacteria in yogurt could end vaginal yeast infections. Certain good bacteria naturally live in this part of your body and help limit the growth of yeast here. When everything works, you have a harmonious balance of bacteria and yeast. But when the bacteria die off, the yeast multiply rapidly, resulting in a yeast infection. Yogurt can help replenish some of those good bacteria. Eating a cup of yogurt each day could be just the thing to prevent or treat vaginal yeast infections, especially if you are prone to them or taking a round of antibiotics. Your bones will thank you, too, since an 8-ounce serving provides about one-third of your daily dose of calcium. Buy yogurt with the "Live and Active Cultures" seal on the carton or the words "active," "live," or "viable" cultures on its label.

12 **Steer clear with asparagus.** Folate, a B vitamin, not only protects you from vaginitis — it may also cut your risk of cervical cancer. Researchers think low levels of folate may leave tissues more vulnerable to cancer-causing substances. Reap the benefits of this B vitamin by eating more asparagus, an excellent source of folate. Perk up wilted asparagus or keep a new bunch fresh by cutting half an inch off the bottom of the stalk. Then stand the stalks in an inch of warm water, and avoid getting the tips wet.

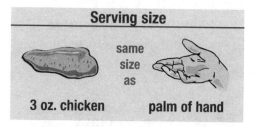

Serving size

same size as

3 oz. chicken · palm of hand

13 **Don't chicken out on zinc.** About half of all adult women in the United States get substantially less than the recommended 8 milligrams (mg) a day of zinc. That's bad news for them because this mineral may help fight yeast infections. Chicken, seafood, legumes, and whole grains are all excellent sources of zinc.

Watch out!

Can't find relief from painful fibrocystic breasts? You may have to cut caffeine completely out of your diet — no more coffee, chocolate, caffeinated sodas, or pain relievers made with caffeine. Wean yourself off gradually, and abstain from caffeine for four months. You may notice fewer, smaller, or less painful lumps. Some women may not see any change.

14 **Go nuts for mixed nuts.** Women who suffer from chronic vaginitis tend to have low levels of the mineral selenium. Experts aren't sure how this mineral helps fight off infections, but you can benefit from its protection right away. Grab a handful of nuts and start munching. Just one ounce of oil-roasted mixed nuts gives you more than twice your recommended daily dose of selenium. Look for this mineral in other unprocessed foods, too, like fresh fruits, vegetables, and whole grains.

15 **Carve up a pumpkin.** This orange icon of Halloween isn't just for autumn holidays. Pumpkins boast loads of alpha and beta carotene, which your body turns into vitamin A. This nutrient helps battle bothersome vaginal infections as well as dry skin during menopause. The cells lining the vagina act as a protective barrier against bacteria and other outside organisms, so it's especially important to keep them healthy. Otherwise, bacteria can get past these defenses and cause infection. Vitamin A helps these cells stay healthy. Bake a pumpkin pie for a sweet slice of beta carotene. Bright yellow and orange vegetables such as carrots and sweet potatoes are also excellent sources, as are dark green veggies like spinach.

End benign breast disorders

Limit the fat in your diet, and you may close the book on breast disorders. Women who suffer from benign breast disorders tend to eat foods higher in fat and calories than those who don't. Saturated fat in meat and dairy products could be a particular culprit. All the extra fat and calories may cause your body to produce more hormones, which in turn trigger the development of lumps and cysts in breast tissue. Choose lean meats and low-fat dairy products, and limit fat calories.

Animal foods such as eggs and fortified dairy products deliver vitamin A itself.

16 **Rein in pain with trout.** Eating foods filled with heart-healthy omega-3 fats may ease the discomfort of fibrocystic breast disease. Women with this condition develop harmless but painful fluid-filled cysts in their breasts. Cold water fish like trout and salmon are fantastic sources of omega-3. Bake or broil an occasional filet, or shred cooked salmon and serve over a cold salad.

Men's health matters

17 foods to recharge and renew

Odds are, if you're a man you will face a prostate problem some time in your life. When most men hit middle age, their prostate begins to grow.

An enlarged prostate can contribute to erectile dysfunction (ED), or cause a noncancerous condition known as benign prostatic hyperplasia (BPH) where you have trouble urinating. Then again, some men develop prostatitis, an extremely painful, inflamed infection of the prostate. Worse yet, many men will face prostate cancer, the second most common cancer among men in the United States.

But prostate problems don't have to be a normal part of aging for men. The nutrients in certain foods can help you beat the odds and prevent or even treat BPH, prostatitis, erectile dysfunction, and cancer.

Chances are, you eat some of these foods, like cauliflower, already. Maybe you just need more. Read on to find out what to eat, how much, and how to prepare it to ward off prostate problems.

1 **Crack open a crab.** The mineral zinc may help shrink enlarged prostates or reduce inflammation from chronic prostatitis — and shellfish like crabs are simply stuffed with it. Zinc is especially important for a healthy prostate. This gland contains up to 10 times the zinc found in other areas of your body, and some studies suggest building more zinc into your diet could help alleviate benign prostatic hyperplasia (BPH). Men should aim to meet their recommended dietary allowance (RDA) of 11 milligrams (mg) of zinc every day. Food is the safest source since supplements can cause zinc toxicity. A single serving of crab starts you off with about 7 mg of this mineral.

2 **Get the scoop on pumpkin seeds.** They're pumped up with zinc, too, which could explain why people have used them for centuries as a folk remedy for prostate problems. In fact, Middle Eastern men in some countries munch a handful of pumpkin seeds every day to prevent BPH. These seeds also contain chemicals that stop your body from turning the hormone testosterone into dihydrotestosterone, which may contribute to an enlarged prostate. Shop for dried pumpkin seeds at your local whole foods or health food store, or make your own from the family jack-o-lantern.

Saw palmetto fails test

More than two million men in the U.S. alone treat their BPH with the herb saw palmetto. Even doctors agreed it might actually help. But a new study published in the *New England Journal of Medicine* has now cast doubt. Out of 225 men, half took 160 milligrams of saw palmetto extract and half took a placebo. After one year, the two groups saw no difference in prostate size, ability to urinate, or quality of life. The researchers concluded that the famous herb worked no better than placebo for treating BPH.

3 **Maximize zinc with chicken.** Eating more zinc is all well and good, but your body needs other nutrients to put it to work protecting the prostate. Vitamin B6, or pyridoxine, is one of them. Men over the age of 50 need at least 1.7 mg of B6 daily, and poultry puts you on your way. A lean cut of chicken breast dishes up more than a third of that amount. Serve it with a helping of black beans for an extra side of zinc.

4 **Just add water.** Something as simple as drinking more water could give you significant relief from prostate pain, especially prostatitis. Men with prostate problems may try to drink less fluid to avoid the frequent, urgent need to urinate. But dehydrating your body can actually cause urine to become too concentrated, setting the stage for a bladder infection. Instead of drinking less, drink smarter. Make water your beverage of choice for the most benefit from your fluids.

5 **Guzzle some cranberry juice.** These tart little berries can sweep away bacteria to help prevent infections in your bladder and prostate. Cranberry juice has been used for centuries as a folk remedy to ward off urinary tract infections (UTIs). Compounds in the berries called proanthocyanidins seem to keep infection-causing bacteria such as *Escherichia coli* (*E. coli*) — the cause of 80 percent of bacterial prostatitis cases — from clinging to the walls of the urinary tract. Opinions vary on how much juice you should drink to

Watch out!

Remember, cranberries can help prevent — but not necessarily treat — bacterial infections, and you may not see results for four to eight weeks. Talk to your doctor before trying this treatment if you take the drug warfarin or have a history of oxalate kidney stones.

Put the brakes on prostate cancer

The next big breakthrough could be sitting in your medicine cabinet. Taking a daily aspirin or ibuprofen could cut your risk of prostate cancer in half. These non-steroidal anti-inflammatory drugs (NSAIDs) seem to slow tumor growth, cause cancer cells to self-destruct, plus boost the body's natural anti-cancer defenses. Experts say it's too early to tell what dose might offer the most protection, but men already taking these drugs to prevent a heart attack or treat arthritis might enjoy a nice bonus. Long-term use of NSAIDs carries serious side effects, so talk to your doctor before taking them regularly.

reap this benefit, ranging anywhere from 3 to 16 ounces daily. Decide what's right for you, and give it a try.

6 Pour soy milk in your cereal. Foods made from soybeans may guard against prostate inflammation. Soy seems to block the production of testosterone linked to prostatitis. In a lab study, rats that were deprived of soy for 11 weeks developed severe prostate inflammation. This tiny bean may prevent prostate cancer, too. Both Chinese and Japanese men are less likely to develop this disease than men in other parts of the world, and experts suspect at least part of that protection could come from eating lots of soy products. Enjoy your breakfast cereal with half soy milk and half regular milk, and add cubed, extra firm tofu to stir-fry. Or maybe tempeh is more your style. This Japanese delicacy comes in a firmer, cake-like form and has a more distinct taste than tofu. Grill it, stir-fry it, or serve it plain or as a shish kebab.

7 **Bite into an apple.** A plant compound called quercetin could improve prostatitis and stop the growth of cancer cells. Quercetin is a flavonoid, a type of phytochemical found in apples, buckwheat, tea, red onions, and citrus fruits that seems to dampen inflammation and fight bacteria as well as cancer. In particular, this compound may improve prostatitis symptoms in some men by quelling prostate inflammation. Quercetin may also prevent prostate cancer by preventing the growth of tumor cells. Munch several apples a week, enjoy a cup of tea, and flip a few buckwheat pancakes for a healthy dose of quercetin.

8 **Snack on cauliflower.** You could slash your prostate cancer risk 41 percent just by lunching on cauliflower at least three times a week. This and other cruciferous vegetables such as broccoli and cabbage contain phytonutrients called glucosinolates. These compounds help stimulate your body to release enzymes that shut down cancer-causing substances. Once neutralized, these dangerous compounds get flushed out of your body before they cause harm. Lightly steam, stir-fry, or eat these veggies raw for the most nutritional punch.

TIP
Buying

Shop for fish instead of red meat to cut out harmful saturated fat and maybe prevent prostate cancer. Men who frequently eat fish are up to three times less likely to get prostate cancer than those who rarely or never eat it. For the biggest bite out of cancer, choose fish rich in "good" omega-3 fats, like salmon, herring, and mackerel.

9 **Steam up some broccoli.** Just eating plenty of vegetables — at least 24 servings each week — could cut your risk of prostate cancer 35 percent, compared to people who eat less than 14 servings weekly. That's what researchers recently discovered. But not just any veggie will do. Out of all the vegetables in this study, brassicas — broccoli, cauliflower, brussels sprouts, kohlrabi, and cabbage — stood out. These cruciferous vegetables contain sulfurophanes, chemical compounds that nix cancer-causing agents before they can harm your cells. Eating broccoli and other brassicas three or more times a week can lower your risk of prostate cancer more than 40 percent. Plus, broccoli is an excellent source of both fiber and vitamin C. Serve it up lightly steamed, or snack on it raw.

TIP
Buying

Cool off on a hot summer day with a chilled-out treat. Puree some seedless watermelon and pour it into an ice cube tray. Freeze, then plop these sweet-tasting cubes into any summer drink. Watermelon is loaded with lycopene, so both your beverage and your prostate will thank you.

10 **Pour on tomato sauce.** Eating at least 10 servings of tomato-based products a week slashed men's risk of prostate cancer by 45 percent in a Harvard University study. A Yale study found similar results. The hero here may be lycopene, a type of plant compound called a carotenoid that gives tomatoes, papaya, pink grapefruit, and watermelon their red color. Lycopene is a powerful antioxidant that may prevent some of the cell damage that leads to cancer, especially in the prostate. Scientists believe other natural compounds in tomatoes team up with lycopene to maximize its cancer-fighting power.

Cooked tomato products like ketchup and tomato sauce seem to serve up more cancer protection than raw tomatoes. Chopping and cooking these vegetables seems to break down the cell walls, making it easier for your body to absorb the nutrients.

11 **Beat cancer odds with apricots.**
Brightly colored vegetables and fruits, like apricots, are not only beautiful — they're also loaded with beta carotene, another carotenoid that could protect you from prostate cancer. Men with low levels of beta carotene in their blood are 45 percent more likely to develop this disease than those with healthy high levels. Apricots contain lycopene, too, for a double dose of cancer protection. Beef up your defenses and shop for fresh or dried apricots at your supermarket.

Here's to your health

In a recent study, men who drank one or two drinks a day cut their risk of impotence by one-third compared with those who drank more often or not at all. It appears moderation is the key.

12 **Break off a stalk of celery.** This healthful snack is rich in selenium, a trace mineral studies say may inhibit the growth of prostate cells. Selenium is also an antioxidant that protects your cells and tissues from oxidation, which sets the stage for cancer. Add up these benefits, and you get top-notch protection from prostate cancer. Aim at least for the RDA of 55 micrograms daily. You can easily meet this goal by eating fresh, unprocessed foods like celery every day, and cutting back on sugar. High-sugar diets contribute to selenium deficiency. Mushrooms, seafood, cabbage, and broccoli are also good sources. Cook them lightly to preserve the most selenium. Boiling vegetables can cut their selenium content almost in half.

13 **Munch on crunchy walnuts.** This little nut contains one of the biggest natural stores of ellagic acid, a flavonoid in plants that fights cancerous tumors. So a few walnuts a day could safeguard your prostate. Those are the findings from the University of Massachusetts Medical School, which examined the link between prostate cancer and diet in 59 countries. Certain foods, including nuts, cereal, and grains seemed to protect against this deadly disease. Sprinkle a few walnuts on your salad, or munch a handful instead of potato chips. Remember, nuts are still high in fat, albeit the good kind, so don't go overboard if you're watching your weight.

Vegetable Viagra?

People once believed artichokes were powerful aphrodisiacs. Doctors commonly prescribed them like a vegetable Viagra for male patients long before such a drug existed. Considering the many other benefits of artichokes, testing this remedy for yourself certainly won't hurt.

14 **Cook with canola oil.** What you eat matters because food is medicine. Take the kinds of fat you cook with. Experts have known monounsaturated fatty acids (MUFAs) are good for your heart, but now they believe MUFAs also protect your prostate. People who eat at least one teaspoon of MUFA-packed oils daily — such as canola, olive, or peanut oil — have half the risk of prostate cancer as people who don't eat MUFA foods. Turn over a new leaf, and choose to cook with canola instead of corn, soybean, cottonseed, or safflower oils.

15 **Make a sandwich with whole-wheat bread.** Clogged arteries and high cholesterol are often intimately linked to erectile dysfunction (ED). Men with total cholesterol above 240 mg/dl are twice as likely to have trouble achieving or maintaining an erection as men whose cholesterol levels are below 180 mg/dl. One of the simplest solutions is to eat more fiber. Fiber helps bind up cholesterol in your intestines and sweep it out of your body before it gets absorbed into your bloodstream. For more fiber, look no further than whole grains. Check the fiber content of cereals, and read the ingredient label of pastas, breads, and other foods carefully. Those made from whole grains should list ingredients such as whole oats, whole wheat, whole rye, cracked wheat, or graham flour as the first ingredient.

16 **Sip some pomegranate juice.** New research suggests drinking pomegranate juice could prevent erectile dysfunction (ED). A natural body process called oxidation can, over time, damage the heart, blood vessels, and other tissue. This, in turn, can contribute to ED. Fortunately, nature makes a natural remedy. Many fruits and vegetables contain antioxidants, plant compounds that neutralize

Chocolate: igniting passion for centuries

Chocolate bars are a popular treat today, but long ago people used to drink chocolate in liquid form as a sweet aphrodisiac, sometimes with spices added. Legend has it the Aztec emperor Montezuma drank 50 cups a day for virility, and Casanova always had some chocolate before meeting with ladies. Chocolate could work as well today as it did back then. It contains amphetamine-like chemicals that mimic the brain chemistry of someone in love. Combine that with a quick energy boost from the sugar, and you've got a recipe for romance.

free radicals — the bad boys behind oxidation — before they damage your cells. Pomegranate juice is packed with powerful antioxidants known as polyphenols. In fact, it contains more polyphenols than green tea; red wine; or cranberry, orange, or blueberry juice. Researchers who tested pomegranate juice on rabbits with ED say it increased penile blood flow and relaxed muscles, and they believe drinking it regularly could help men prevent ED. This study used the brand POM Wonderful, made of 100 percent pomegranate juice.

17 **Have a bowl of black bean soup.** Black beans are gold mines of a protein known as L-arginine that seems to increase blood flow to the penis for better erections. In one small study, one-third of men with ED who ate 5 grams of L-arginine daily — the equivalent of 5 cups of cooked black beans — for six weeks were able to have normal erections again. Five cups of beans may be a little extreme, but why not add a serving or two each day and see if you notice a natural difference. Worried about gas? Change the water after soaking the beans, or add a few drops of Beano, an anti-gas remedy, to cooked beans before eating.

Sources

A citrus a day keeps the doctor away, Commonwealth Scientific & Industrial Research Organization <http://www.csiro.au/index.asp> retrieved Feb. 2, 2006

A Field Guide to Buying Organic, Bantam Dell, New York, 2005

A Food Labeling Guide — Appendix C, U.S. Food and Drug Administration/Center for Food Safety and Applied Nutrition <www.cfsan.fda.gov/~dms/flg-6c.html> retrieved Feb. 22, 2006

About Nausea and Vomiting, Cleveland Clinic Health Information Center <http://www.clevelandclinic.org/health/health-info/docs/1800/1810.asp?index=8106> retrieved March 14, 2005

ACS Cancer Detection Guidelines, American Cancer Society <http://www.cancer.org/docroot/PED/content/PED_2_3X_ACS_Cancer_Detection_Guidelines_36.asp?sitearea=PED> retrieved Feb. 6, 2006

Advances in Food and Nutrition Research (45:1-60)

Alimentary Pharmacology and Therapeutics (22,9:795)

All About Brussels Sprouts, Ocean Mist Farms, Inc. <www.oceanmist.com> retrieved Aug. 10, 2005

Allergy (55,12:1184)

Almond Milk, A Boke of Gode Cookery Recipes <www.godecookery.com> retrieved Jan. 30, 2006

Sources

Almonds, daily exercise keep brain healthy, USA Today, Nov. 14, 2006

Alternative Medicine Review (8,3:247 and 8,3:284)

Alzheimer's & Dementia: The Journal of the Alzheimer's Association (1,1:11)

American Dietetic Association Complete Food and Nutrition Guide, 2nd edition, John Wiley & Sons, Hoboken, N.J., 2002

American Dry Bean Board — Bean Basics
<http://www.americanbean.org/BeanBasics/Home.htm> retrieved Sept. 22, 2005

American Family Physician (70,1:133; 71,7:1375; and 72,1:103)

American Journal of Cardiology (96,6:810)

American Journal of Clinical Nutrition (53,5:1259; 77,3:600; 79,1:70; 79,6:935; 79,6 Suppl:1158S; 80,2:396; 80,6:1508; 81,2:508; 81,4:773; 81,4:934; 81.5:1045; 81,6:1417; and 82,3:575)

American Journal of Epidemiology (145,1:42; and 161,10:948)

American Journal of Gastroenterology (100,7:1539)

American Journal of Medicine (117,3:169)

American Journal of Preventive Medicine (29,4:302)

American Journal of Public Health (96,2:9)

American Physiological Society news release (April 3, 2005)

Annals of Allergy, Asthma, & Immunology (95,1:4; and 94,4:480)

Annals of Internal Medicine (132,8:680; 141,11:846; 142,6:144; 142,6:469; and 143,1:1)

Sources

Annals of Nutrition and Metabolism (49,3:141)

Annals of Oncology (16,3:359)

Annals of the Rheumatic Diseases (63,7:843)

Antimicrobial Phytochemicals in Thompson Seedless Raisins (Vitis vinifera L.) Inhibit Dental Plaque Bacteria, Paper presented at 105th General Meeting of the American Society for Microbiology, June 8, 2005, Atlanta, Ga.

Appetite (43,2:207)

Apples really are good for you, Washington Apple Commission <http://www.bestapples.com/healthy/index.html> retrieved May 2, 2005

Archives of Internal Medicine (164,20:2235; 165,9:997; 165,16:1890; 165,22:2683; and 165,4:393)

Archives of Neurology (62:1)

Archives of Ophthalmology (122,6:883; and 123,4:517)

Archives of Oral Biology (50,7:645)

Archives of Otolaryngology — Head & Neck Surgery (130,12:1381)

Arthritis & Rheumatism (50,6:1822; and 50:1,72)

Asia Pacific Journal of Clinical Nutrition (13:S74)

Atkins Advantage Products, Atkins Nutritionals, Inc. <www.atkins.com>

B vitamins do not protect hearts, BBC NEWS <http://news.bbc.co.uk/go/pr/fr/-/1/hi/health/4218186.stm> retrieved Sept. 29, 2005

Sources

Barley Products, National Barley Foods Council, www.barleyfoods.org retrieved Dec. 23, 2005

BENECOL Smart Chews and Spreads, BENECOL <http://www.benecol.com/products/index.jhtml> retrieved Nov. 28, 2005

Beta-cryptoxanthin, The World's Healthiest Foods <www.whfoods.org> retrieved Dec. 5, 2005

Biochimica et Biophysica Acta (1581,3:89)

Biofactors (13,1-4:265)

Biological Psychiatry (57,4:343)

Biological Trace Element Research (66:1-3,299)

BMC Psychiatry (4,1:36)

BMC Women's Health (5,1:9)

Boosting Calcium with Nonfat Dry Milk, The Pennsylvania State University Extension Services <http://pubs.cas.psu.edu/FreePubs> retrieved Feb. 11, 2000

Boron content of some common foods, GreenFacts.org ToolBox <www.greenfacts.org> retrieved Dec. 2, 2005

Bowe's & Church's Food Values of Portions Commonly Used, 18th Edition, Lippincott Williams & Wilkins, Baltimore, Md., 2004

Brain Foods, AskDrSears.com <http://askdrsears.com/html/4/t040400.asp#T040405> retrieved Nov. 8, 2005

British Journal of Cancer (90,1:128)

Sources

British Journal of Community Nursing (8,12:S14)

British Journal of Dentistry (199,4:213)

British Journal of Nutrition (80,4:S209; 82,2:125; 86,2:233; 91,1:141; and 91,6:991)

British Medical Journal (317,7174:1683)

Broccoli sprout extracts inhibit bladder cancer cell proliferation, Paper presented at: 2005 Institute of Food Technologists Annual Meeting; July 15-20, 2005; New Orleans, La.

Brown Rice Basics, USA Rice Federation <http://www.usarice.com> retrieved Aug. 4, 2005

Calcium good for more than strong bones, USA Today (133,2721:10)

Canadian Family Physician (49,2:168)

Canadian Journal of Gastroenterology (14,6:521)

Canadian Medical Association Journal (173,9:1043)

Cancer (104,4:879)

Cancer Epidemiology Biomarkers and Prevention (14,1:126 and 14,3:740)

Cancer Research (65,18:8339 and 65,18:8548)

Cancer Science (96,1:1)

Celery, The World's Healthiest Foods <www.whfoods.org> retrieved Jan. 25, 2006

Chest (118,4:1150 and 129,1S:249S)

Sources

Chicago Sun-Times (Sept. 7, 2005)

Childhood exposure to second-hand smoke has long-lasting effects: Fruit fiber may help, Medical News Today <http://www.medicalnewstoday.com/printerfriendlynews.php?newsid=29890> retrieved Sept. 2, 2005

Circulation (105,16:1897)

Claims That Can Be Made for Conventional Foods and Dietary Supplements, U.S. Food and Drug Administration/Center for Food Safety and Applied Nutrition <www.cfsan.fda.gov/~dms/hclaims.html> retrieved Feb. 22, 2006

Clinical Diabetes (19,1:4)

Clinical Gastroenterology and Hepatology (3,4:358)

Clinical Infectious Diseases (40:807)

Cook's Illustrated (68:31)

Cooking Safely in the Microwave Oven, USDA Food Safety and Inspection Service <www.foodsafety.gov/~fsg/fs-mwave.html> retrieved Feb. 8, 2006

Cranberries, The World's Healthiest Foods <http://www.whfoods.com/genpage.php?tname=foodspice&dbid=145> retrieved May 31, 2005

Critical Reviews in Food Science and Nutrition (41,4:251)

Crohns & Colitis Foundation of America <www.ccfa.org> retrieved April 4, 2005

Sources

Crohns Disease, Johns Hopkins Medical Institutions Gastroenterology & Hepatology Resource Center <http://hopkins-gi.nts.jhu.edu/pages/latin/templates/index.cfm?pg=disease1&organ=6&disease=21&lang_id=1> retrieved March 28, 2005

Cuisine at Home (1,50:39 and 1,52:4)

Depression, National Institute of Mental Health <www.nimh.nih.gov/healthinformation/depressionmenu.cfm> retrieved Oct. 12, 2005

Dermatologic Surgery (31,7 Pt 2:814)

Diabetes and Metabolism (29,6:635)

Diabetes Care (27,10:2491 and 27,1:281)

Dietary Guidelines for Americans, 6th Edition, U.S. Department of Health and Human Services and U.S. Department of Agriculture, Washington, D.C., January 2005

Dietary Reference Intakes, National Academy Press, Washington, 2002

Digestive Health & Nutrition (July/August 2005)

Drug Interactions: Factors Affecting Response to Drugs, Merck Manual Home Edition <www.merck.com/mmhe/sec02/ch013/ch013c.html>

Drugs under Experimental and Clinical Research (25,5:219; 25,6:281; and 28,2-3:49)

Eating Well as We Age, U.S. Food and Drug Administration, Department of Health and Human Services, Rockville, Md.

Edible and Medicinal Mushrooms: Chemistry and Biological Effects, Paper presented at The 230th American Chemical Society National Meeting, Aug 28-Sept. 1, 2005, Washington, D.C.

Sources

Effects of Yoghurt on the Human Oral Microbiota and Halitosis, Paper presented at: The IADR/AADR/CADR 83rd General Session, March 9-12 2005, Baltimore, Md.

Encyclopedia of Nutrition and Good Health, Facts and Comparisons, Inc, New York, 2003

Encyclopedia of the Digestive System and Digestive Disorders, Facts on File, Inc., New York, 2004

Endocrinology (145,9:4366)

Energy bars, unwrapped, ConsumerReports.org <www.consumerreports.org> retrieved Sept. 2, 2003

Environmental Nutrition (May 2002, February 2003, November 2003, January 2004, February 2004, May 2004, October 2004, February 2005, and 25,2:2)

European Food Research and Technology (215,4:310)

European Journal of Clinical Nutrition (58,11:1443 and 59,3:441)

Expert Report Summary, American Institute for Cancer Research <http://www.aicr.org/research/report_summary.lasso> retrieved Sept. 8, 2005

Facts about Asparagus, Michigan Asparagus Advisory Board <www.asparagus.org> retrieved Feb. 2, 2006

Family Practice News (35,14)

Fiber Facts: Soluble Fiber & Heart Disease, American Dietetic Association <www.eatright.org> retrieved Nov. 13, 2002

Sources

Fiber, University of Maryland Medical Center Home Medical Reference
<http://www.umm.edu/altmed/ConsSupplements/Fibercs.html>
retrieved Nov. 16, 2005

Flax — A health and Nutrition Primer, Flax Council of Canada
<www.flaxcouncil.ca> retrieved Feb. 6, 2006

Food and Drug Interactions, National Consumers League, 1701 K
Street, NW, Suite 1200, Washington, D.C. 20006

Food and Mood: the complete guide to eating well and feeling your best,
Henry Holt and Company, Inc., New York, 1995

Food Interactions: Factors Affecting Response to Drugs, Merck Manual
Home Edition <www.merck.com/mmhe/sec02/ch013/ch013e.html>

Foodborne Diseases, National Institute of Allergy and Infectious
Diseases <http://www.niaid.nih.gov/factsheets/foodbornedis.htm>
retrieved Feb. 16, 2005

Free Radical Biology & Medicine (37,9:1351)

Frequently Asked Questions, Pennsylvania Nut Growers Association
<www.pnga.net/faq.html> retrieved Aug. 9, 2005

Fresh Cherries May help Arthritis Sufferers, Agricultural Research, May 2004

Fruit of the Month — Apricots, Centers for Disease Control and
Prevention <http://www.cdc.gov/nccdphp/dnpa/5aday/month/apri-
cot.htm> retrieved July 28, 2005

Fruit of the Month — Kiwi, Centers for Disease Control and Prevention
<www.cdc.gov/nccdphp/dnpa/5aday/month/pdfs/Kiwi.pdf> retrieved
June 21, 2005

Fun facts/papayas, Dole 5 A Day <wwwdole5aday.com> retrieved
June 3, 2005

Sources

Gene Therapy (Dec. 1, 2005)

General Dentistry (52,4:308 and 53,1:73)

Get on the Grain Train, Center for Nutrition Policy and Promotion, U.S. Department of Agriculture, Home and Garden Bulletin No. 267-2

Gluten Free Diet, For Celiac Sprue — Digestion and digestive-related information, MedicineNet.com <http://www.medicinenet.com/script/main/art.asp?articlekey=21462> retrieved June 10, 2005

Grains of Truth about ... Bulgur, Wheat Foods Council <www.wheatfoods.org> retrieved Sept. 1, 2005

Green tea suggests cancer cure, Medline Plus <www.nim.nih.gov> retrieved July 21, 2005

Growing Older, Eating Better, Federal Citizen Information Center <www.pueblo.gsa.gov/cic_text/food/grow_old/grow_old.htm> retrieved June 24, 2005

Gut (53,10:1479 and 54,1:11)

Herring Processing, Gulf of Maine Research Institute <www.gma.org> retrieved Jan. 9, 2006

Honey in Beauty/Personal Care, National Honey Board <http://www.nhb.org/health/MedFactSheets.html> retrieved Sep. 17, 2004

Hong Kong Medical Journal (10,6:414)

Human Reproduction (20,8:2190)

Hypertension (46,2:398)

Sources

IFSCC Magazine (8,1:2)

Indiana University news release (June 8, 2005)

Inflammatory Bowel Disease (11,4:360)

Inflammatory Bowel Disease, The American College of Gastroenterology <www.acg.gi.org> retrieved April 11, 2005

Integrative Medicine (4,1:20)

International Code of Botanical Nomenclature (III,2,18.5)

International Journal of Cancer (114,4:653)

International Journal of Food Microbiology (99,3:257)

International Journal of Obesity and Related Metabolic Disorders (28,12:1569 and 29,4:391)

Investigative Ophthalmology & Visual Science (46,6:2092)

Journal of Advanced Nursing (49,3:234)

Journal of Agricultural and Food Chemistry (50,10:3050; 51,25:7287; 52,1:135; 52,25:7514; 52,26:8151; 52,6:1688; 53,13:5461; 53,9:3408; and 54,1:243)

Journal of Antimicrobial Chemotherapy (54,1:86)

Journal of Applied Physiology (93,4:1227)

Journal of Biological Chemistry (280,45:37377)

Journal of Bone and Mineral Research (20,1:152)

Journal of Clinical Endocrinology and Metabolism (89,3:1217)

Sources

Journal of Clinical Pharmacology (45,10:1153)

Journal of Dental Research (83,7:518)

Journal of Dentistry (31,4:241)

Journal of Food Science (69,9:C702)

Journal of Hypertension (23,3;475)

Journal of Medicinal Food (7,1:100)

Journal of Neuroinflammation (2:8)

Journal of Neuroscience (25,38:8807)

Journal of Nutrition (129,3:751; 133,11:3598; 134,8:1874; 134,12:3225; 135,10:2320; 135,3:592; and 135,9:2096)

Journal of Pharmacological Sciences (95,2:158)

Journal of the American Academy of Dermatology (47,5:709)

Journal of the American College of Nutrition (18,1:43 and 24,1:44)

Journal of the American Dietetic Association (87,9:1164 and 99,3:335)

Journal of the American Geriatric Society (53,3:381 and 53,3;381)

Journal of the American Medical Association (294,10:1255)

Journal of the American Medical Association (293,4:455; 294,1:32; 294,1:97; and 294,24:3101)

Journal of the International Academy of Periodontology (6,2:63)

Journal of the Science of Food and Agriculture (83,14:1511 and 86,1:18)

Sources

Journal of Urology (174,1:386)

Journal of Visual Impairment and Blindness (99,11:725)

Journal of Women's Health & Gender-based Medicine (11,1:61)

Lancet (355,9198:134 and 366,9496:1558)

Life Sciences (73,13:1683)

Lipids (39,2:161)

Live the rural life, avoid asthma? WebMD <http://my.webmd.com/content/article/113/110696?src=RSS_PUBLIC> retrieved Oct. 14, 2005

Macular Degeneration Gene Discovered, Aging Eye Times <www.aging-eye.net/mainnews/gene.php> retrieved Jan. 4, 2006

Make The Switch To Yogurt — There's No Substitute for It, AboutYogurt.com <http://www.aboutyogurt.com/recipes/substitutionTips.asp> retrieved Aug. 16, 2005

Mars offers cholesterol-lowering chocolate bars, Nutra Ingredients USA <http://www.nutraingredients-usa.com/news/printNewsBis.asp?id=62557> retrieved Sept. 15, 2005

Medicine & Science in Sports & Exercise (34,11:1757 and 37:904)

Menopause (12,6:755)

Mercury Levels in Commercial Fish and Shellfish, U.S. Department of Health and Human Services and U.S. Environmental Protection Agency <www.cfsan.fda.gov/~frf/sea-mehg.html> retrieved Feb. 14, 2006

Miracle Health Claims: Add a Dose of Skepticism, Federal Trade Commission <www.ftc.gov/bcp/conline/pubs/health/frdheal.htm> retrieved Feb. 22, 2006

Sources

Molecular Expressions: Phytochemical Gallery — Butyl Phthalide, Florida State University <http://micro.magnet.fsu.edu> retrieved Jan. 25, 2006

More Chicken Soup & Other Folk Remedies, Ballantine Books, New York, 1986

MyPyramid.gov, United States Department of Agriculture <www.mypyramid.gov> retrieved Dec. 19, 2005

National Barley Foods Council <www.barleyfoods.org> retrieved Aug. 5, 2005

National Cancer Institute 5 A Day: Tips, National Cancer Institute <www.5aday.gov> retrieved Aug. 1, 2005

Natural Products Encyclopedia <www.consumerlab.com> retrieved June 2, 2005

Nature (437,7055:45)

Neurology (63,12:2240 and 64,5:817)

New England Journal of Medicine (350,11:1093; 352,22:2271; and 354,6:557)

New York Times (Sept. 16, 2005)

Newer Knowledge of Dairy Foods: Milk, National Dairy Council <http://www.nationaldairycouncil.org/NationalDairyCouncil/Nutritio n/Products/milkPage5.htm> retrieved April 20, 2005

NOW Foods — Rice Bran <http://www.nowfoods.com/?action=itemde-tail&item_id=4019&F=1> retrieved Jan. 20, 2005

Nursing Standard (18,48:38)

Nutrient-Drug Interactions and Food, Colorado State University Cooperative Extension <www.ext.colostate.edu/pubs/foodnut/09361.html#top> retrieved June 29, 2005

Nutrition & the M.D. (30,10:8)

Nutrition (19,3:253)

Nutrition and Cancer (51,2:207)

Nutrition Concepts and Controversies, 10th edition, Thomson Wadsworth, Belmont, Calif., 2006

Nutrition Fact Sheet: Water, Feinberg School of Medicine, Northwestern University <www.feinberg.northwestern.edu/nutrition/factsheets/water.html> retrieved Feb. 17, 2006

Nutrition Facts & Calorie Counter, NutritionData.com <www.nutritiondata.com> retrieved Sept. 2, 2005

Nutrition Facts, 100% Pomegranate Juice, POM Wonderful <http://www.pomwonderful.com/100_percent_juice.html> retrieved Feb. 1, 2006

Nutrition Notes, National Barley Foods Council <www.barleyfoods.org> retrieved Aug. 5, 2005

Nutrition Reviews (54,11:S38 and 63,1:1)

Nutrition's Role, The Macular Degeneration Partnership <www.amd.org> retrieved Feb. 16, 2006

NutritionData.com <http://www.nutritiondata.com>

Obstetrics and Gynecology (105,5:1074)

Sources

Oral Microbiology and Immunology (19,2:118)

Osteoporosis Overview, National Institutes of Health Osteoporosis and Related Bone Diseases — National Resource Center, Bethesda, Md.

Periodontal Disease — UMMC, A.D.A.M., Inc.
<http://www.umm.edu/patiented/articles/what_causes_periodontal_disease_000024_3.htm> retrieved Feb. 7, 2006

Physicians Committee for Responsible Medicine news release (May 27, 2000)

Physiological Effects of Dietary Fiber (from Carbohydrates in human nutrition, FAO Food and Nutrition Paper — 66), Food and Agriculture Organization of the United Nations
<http://www.fao.org/docrep/w8079e/w8079e0l.htm> retrieved Jan. 16, 2005

Pinto beans, The World's Healthiest Foods <www.whfoods.com> retrieved Aug. 26, 2005

Potentially Modifiable Risk Factors for Dementia: Evidence from Identical Twins. Paper presented at: Alzheimer's Association International Conference on Prevention of Dementia, Washington, D.C., June 18-21

PowerBar Products <www.powerbar.com>

Prevention, American Obesity Association
<www.obesity.org/prevention/maintaining.shtml> retrieved Aug. 16, 2005

Proceedings of the National Academy of Sciences of the United States of America 2005 (102,41:14813)

Products, The Balance Bar Food Company <www.balance.com>

Pulse (65,43:46)

Sources

Qualified Health Claims Subject to Enforcement Discretion, U.S. Food and Drug Administration/Center for Food Safety and Applied Nutrition <www.cfsan.fda.gov/~dms/qhc-sum.html> retrieved Feb. 22, 2006

Raisins, The World's Healthiest Foods: Eating Healthy <www.whfoods.com> retrieved June 23, 2005

Real Simple (5,4:159)

Researchers Make Colorful Rice <http://www.msnbc.msn.com/id/8410300/> retrieved June 30, 2005

Resources for Home Preserving Pumpkins, National Center for Home Food Preservation <http://www.uga.edu/nchfp/tips/fall/pumpkins.html> retrieved Jan. 20, 2005

Revealing Trans Fats, U.S. Food and Drug Administration <www.pueblo.gsa.gov>

Rheological Properties of Biopolymeric Composites of Cellulosic and Beta-Glucan Hydrocolloidal Gels. United States Department of Agriculture, Agricultural Research Service <www.ars.usda.gov> retrieved Aug. 23, 2005

Salt: The Forgotten Killer, Center for Science in the Public Interest, 1875 Connecticut Ave NW, #300, Washington, D.C. 20009

Sara Lee introduces white bread made with whole grain, Just-Food.com <www.just-food.com/news_details.asp?art=61371&lk=emf> retrieved July 21, 2005

Sauerkraut consumption may fight off breast cancer, Nutraingredients.com <http://www.nutraingredients.com/news/ng.asp?n=63688&m=1FSN N08&idP=2&c=mzwqdgpetgmbhyl)> retrieved Jan. 6, 2006

Science (305,5691:1736)

Sources

Science In Your Shopping Cart, United States Department of Agriculture <www.npa.ars.usda.gov> retrieved July 13, 2005

Science News (166,16:248)

Sports Medicine (33,9:671)

Stroke (36,7:1426)

Swedish Dental Journal (27,1:31)

Sweet Dreams are Made of Cheese, British Cheese Board <http://www.cheeseboard.co.uk/news.cfm?y=y&page_id=2...> retrieved Oct. 3, 2005

The Chicago Tribune (July 6, 2005)

The Encyclopedia of Nutrition and Good Health, 2nd Edition, Facts on File Inc., New York, 2003

The Johns Hopkins White Papers: Diabetes, Medletter Associates, Inc., Redding, Conn., 2005

The Linus Pauling Institute Micronutrient Information Center <http://lpi.oregonstate.edu/infocenter>

The Merck Manual, 16th Edition, Merck & Co., Inc, Rahway, N.J., 1992

The Nobel Foundation press release (Oct. 3, 2005)

The Nutrition Bible, William Morrow and Company, Inc., New York, 1995

The PDR Family Guide to Nutrition and Health, Medical Economics, Montvale, N.J. 1995

Sources

The Protective Effect of Wine Intake on Five Year's Incidence of Cataract, Paper presented at: Association for Research in Vision and Ophthalmology 2005 Annual Meeting; May 4, 2005; Fort Lauderdale, Fla.

The Review of Natural Products, Facts and Comparisons Publishing Group, St. Louis, Mo., 2004

The Saturday Evening Post (276,1:60)

The Unwelcome Dinner Guest: Preventing Foodborne Illness, U.S. Food and Drug Administration <www.fda.gov/fdac/reprints/dinguest.html> retrieved Feb. 8, 2006

The Wall Street Journal (Oct. 14, 2003, D1; March 29, 2005, D4; July 19, 2005, D7; Aug. 30, 2005, D5; and Jan. 10, 2006, D1)

The Washington Post (Feb. 16, 2003)

The Whole Foods Companion, Chelsea Green Publishing Company, White River Junction, Vt., 2004

To remember, don't forget the caffeine <http://abcnews.go.com/Health/print?id=1360863> retrieved Dec. 6, 2005

Tufts Daily, Tufts University School of Nutrition Science and Policy (September 2004)

Turnips, Healthnotes, Inc. <www.publix.com> retrieved Feb. 10, 2006

U.S. Pharmacist (29,8:32)

UMass Dartmouth researcher identifies cancer-fighting cranberry compound, NutraIngredients.com <http://www.umassd.edu/communications/articles/showarticles.cfm?a_key=469> retrieved Dec. 28, 2005

Sources

University of Buffalo news release (June 16, 2002)

University of North Carolina at Chapel Hill news release (Nov. 13, 2005)

USA Rice Federation
<http://www.usarice.com/consumer/presskit.html> retrieved Aug. 24, 2005

USDA National Nutrient Database for Standard Reference, Release 18,
United States Department of Agriculture <www.nal.usda.gov>

USDA News Release (July 26, 2005)

Using the Diabetes Food Pyramid, American Diabetes Association
<www.diabetes.org/nutrition-and-recipes/nutrition/foodpyramid.jsp>
retrieved Jan. 26, 2006

Vitamin B6 (Pyridoxine), University of Maryland Medicine
<www.umm.edu> retrieved Jan. 3, 2005

Wellness Foods A to Z, Rebus, Inc., New York, 2002

What You Need to Know About Mercury in Fish and Shellfish, U.S.
Department of Health and Human Services and U.S. Environmental
Protection Agency <www.cfsan.fda.gov/~dms/admehg3.html>
retrieved Feb. 14, 2006

Who'da thunk it?! Organics go private-label, MSNBC.com
<www.msnbc.msn.com/id/9053689/> retrieved Aug. 24, 2005

*Whole Foods Companion: A Guide for Adventurous Cooks, Curious Shoppers,
and Lovers of Natural Foods,* Chelsea Green Publishing Co., White
River Junction, Vt., 2004

Wiadomosci lekarskie 2004 (57[S1]:233)

Sources

Wild Oats — The Webb Cooks, American Diabetes Association <www.diabetes.org> retrieved Jan. 16, 2006

Winter Squash, Pennsylvania Nutrition Education Network <http://panen.psu.edu/intranet/snap/winter_squash/wintersquash_n ewsletter.pdf> retrieved Jan. 20, 2006

Women's Health & Wellness 2005, Oxmoor House, Inc., Birmingham, Ala., 2004

World Journal of Gastroenterology (9,3:408)

World Journal of Urology (20,5:273)

Yoplait Healthy Heart has plant sterols, Yoplait <http://www.yoplait.com/YHHealthFAQ.htm> retrieved Oct. 12, 2005

Your Health: Nutrition and the Older Adult, Calgary Health Region Learning and Development <http://yourhealth.calgaryhealthregion.ca> retrieved March 22, 2005

Index